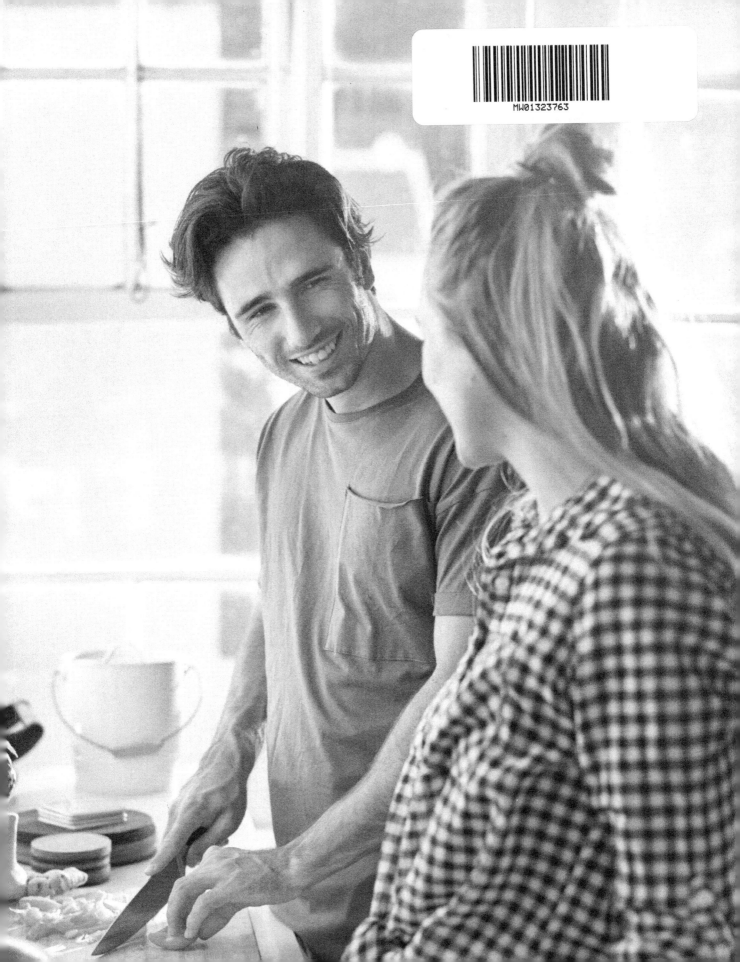

Air Fryer Cookbook for Two

250 Quick & Easy, Perfectly Portioned Recipes.
Fry, Roast, Bake & Grill Your Favorite Meals.

Emily Anderson - 2021 Edition

© Copyright 2021 by Emily Anderson - All rights reserved.

The following Book is reproduced below with the goal of providing information that is as accurate and reliable as possible. Regardless, purchasing this Book can be seen as consent to the fact that both the publisher and the author of this book are in no way experts on the topics discussed within and that any recommendations or suggestions that are made herein are for entertainment purposes only. Professionals should be consulted as needed prior to undertaking any of the action endorsed herein.

This declaration is deemed fair and valid by both the American Bar Association and the Committee of Publishers Association and is legally binding throughout the United States.

Furthermore, the transmission, duplication, or reproduction of any of the following work including specific information will be considered an illegal act irrespective of if it is done electronically or in print. This extends to creating a secondary or tertiary copy of the work or a recorded copy and is only allowed with the express written consent from the Publisher. All additional right reserved.

The information in the following pages is broadly considered a truthful and accurate account of facts and as such, any inattention, use, or misuse of the information in question by the reader will render any resulting actions solely under their purview. There are no scenarios in which the publisher or the original author of this work can be in any fashion deemed liable for any hardship or damages that may befall them after undertaking information described herein.

Additionally, the information in the following pages is intended only for informational purposes and should thus be thought of as universal. As befitting its nature, it is presented without assurance regarding its prolonged validity or interim quality. Trademarks that are mentioned are done without written consent and can in no way be considered an endorsement from the trademark holder.

Contents

Introduction - 5

Benefits of an Air Fryer - 6

Preparing for Two - 7

A Guide to Air Frying – 9

RECIPES

Breakfast - 17

Snacks & Side Dishes - 29

Beef, Pork & Lamb - 36

Poultry - 48

Fish & Seafood - 60

Plant Based - 72

Desserts – 79

Ingredients Index – 87

Conversion Measure – 90

Recipe Index - 93

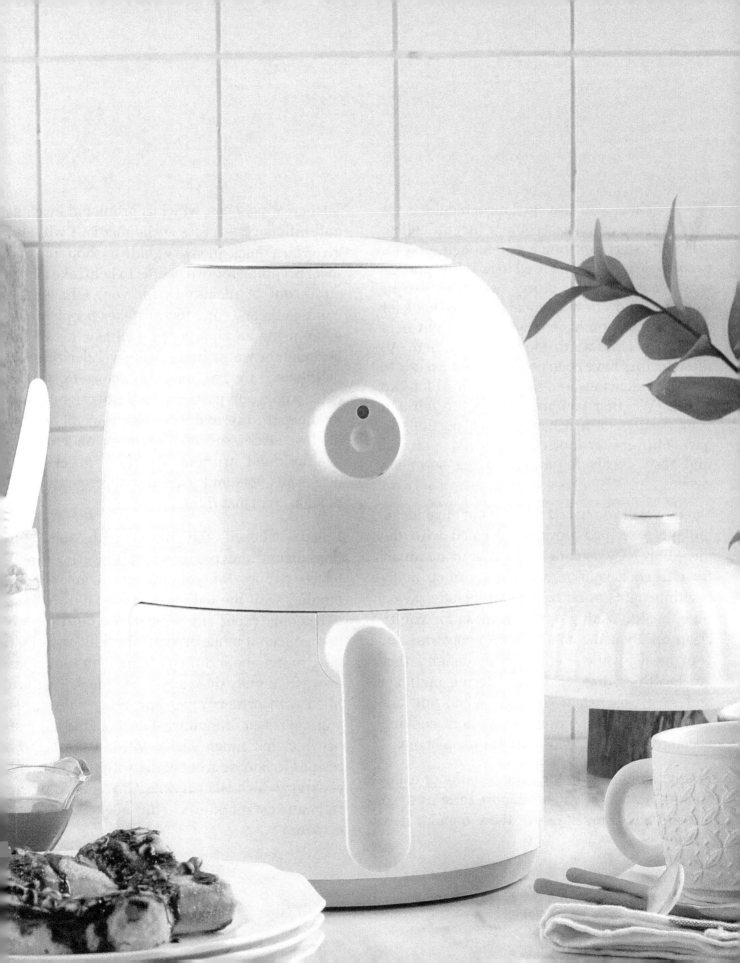

Introduction

When you are no longer cooking for one, it can become a bit difficult to start portioning out enough food for two people if you aren't used to it. While portion size is not your only worry, you may also be wondering how to shop, meal prep, and cook for two. Luckily, you have all you need right here with 250 recipes waiting for you to try them. All these recipes have been portioned out exactly to provide a delicious and satisfying meal for two people. Whether you are cooking for you and your partner or just cooking two portions to have leftovers for lunch the next day, you will find tasty meals to make cooking so much easier.

Not only will you have a whole lot of meal ideas, but these recipes are also designed with the incredibly easy cooking method of using an air fryer to cook your meals. There are so many health benefits of air fryers that include saving time, healthy eating, and less mess for you to clean up. By using an air fryer to cook most of your meals, you can enjoy crispy delights that are healthier than traditional frying methods and save time when cooking. When you are feeding two people, everything about cooking becomes easier with this air fryer recipe book.

Firstly, I will run through the benefits of using an air fryer in case you need more reasons to go out and buy yourself one of these popular new kitchen appliances, which is promoted by chefs and influencers across social media. I will also give you a quick and easy guide to shopping and meal prepping for two people to help take all the stress out of mealtimes for you. I have also compiled a few common mistakes people make when using an air fryer as well as a list of the best and the worst foods to air fry. All of this will be followed by 250 amazing recipes for you to cook with your partner. As a nutritionist and food expert, my goal is to take away all of your kitchen stress so you can focus on enjoying healthy food without the fuss of cleaning numerous pots and pans and never getting the portion sizes just right.

I have chosen the meals with the best ingredients and put together these tried and tested recipes for you because I am all too familiar with the tedious work it takes to feed two people, especially if you have a full-time job or are just not much of a chef. Luckily, you don't have to fret about difficult ingredients anymore or waste money on ready-made meals that are filled with preservatives and other substances you can't even pronounce. Easy cooking has just become that much easier with all these tasty recipes to choose from along with the future of cooking, which is air frying. All you need to eat right and eat on time is in this book. So, let's get cooking!

Benefits of an Air Fryer

Purchasing an air fryer for your kitchen is a worthwhile investment for your cooking needs because of the numerous benefits you will enjoy with your new appliance.

Healthier Cooking Methods

Using an air fryer is a lot healthier than deep frying your favorite fried foods. Not only do you add a lot less oil to your cooking, but the airflow in the air fryer also reduces the amount of oil that is already in the food. Despite the reduction of oil, the appliance still produces crispy foods. The most important health benefit in air fryer cooking is the 90% reduction of acrylamides, which is a cancerous toxin that forms and accumulates when starchy foods are cooked at high temperatures, as is done when deep-frying (*Shubrook, 2020*). However, be careful not to fall into the trap of thinking it's okay to eat a lot of fried food; air frying food means it is still fried food even when prepared with less oil. Luckily, you have this whole recipe book to give you plenty of healthy options for your air fryer.

Reduced Cooking Times

Cooking in an air fryer significantly cuts down your cooking times since you don't have to waste time preheating the oven and you can cook foods directly from frozen. This is an easy option for your frozen prepared meals. Cut out the unhealthy additives by using meal prep techniques rather than buying frozen ready meals, as they contain unnecessary preservatives and ingredients. The rapid circulating hot air and the small size of the air fryer lead to faster cooking times than conventional ovens.

Reduces Mess in the Kitchen

Using an air fryer reduces the need for lots of pots and pans during your cooking since most of your cooking goes into the built-in fryer basket. Most air fryers contain dishwasher-friendly parts, making cleaning so much easier. The lack of oil and the closed basket eliminate any oil splashing around on kitchen surfaces.

Preparing for Two

Preparing meals for two can be quite different if you have become so used to shopping, preparing, and cooking for one. Now you need to work out the right amount of food to prepare and start cooking meals you will both enjoy. Luckily, I have some tips to get you started.

Shopping for Two

Your first order of business is to work out your shopping for two. There is no more rushing to the shop and grabbing a ton of ready-made meals to eat by yourself; you now have someone to enjoy shopping with, and then you both can prepare and cook meals together. Firstly, you will need to decide on the ingredients you both enjoy to base meals around, even if the rest of the meal is different for each person. Here is a basic grocery list to work from, containing a few essential items you should keep on hand at home:

Shopping List for Two			
Monthly	Examples	Weekly	Examples
Meat	Turkey, chicken, beef	Dairy	Milk, cheese, yogurt
Fish	Oily fish like tuna, mackerel, haddock, salmon	Eggs	
Grains	Pasta, rice, oats	Fruit	Apples, bananas, plums
Bread	Whole grain bread, all-purpose flour	Berries	Strawberries, raspberries, blackberries
Oils and fat	Olive oil, coconut oil, butter	Vegetables	Onion, garlic, potatoes, greens, salad veggies
Tinned goods	Beans, legumes, dried fruit, nuts	Frozen fruit	Berries, seasonal fruits
Condiments	Salt, pepper, vinegar, spices	Frozen vegetables	Stir fry veggies, frozen rice

Meal Prep for Two

Meal prep is an easy way to make sure you have healthy meals ready throughout the week for quick and easy meals. When meal prepping for two people, it becomes slightly more challenging to do than for one person, since you have to watch portion sizes—especially if you both don't eat the same amount—and you will need to have a variety to cater for both people. Here are a few quick tips to help you:

Start by meal prepping twice a week; a Sunday and Wednesday are good days to schedule this. Having two sets of meal prep days allows you to have a variety of meals on hand and prevent both of you from getting too bored with the same meals. With regard to meal prepping, this method is more manageable so you don't feel overwhelmed with prepping too much at once.

You can also opt for a buffet-style meal prep where you prep and freeze ingredients separately. So, when it comes to mealtimes, both of you can choose the different elements you want in your dish. This is also helpful if you are catering to different diet preferences such as vegetarianism or veganism. You can have the starches and veggies prepared together with two separate proteins for the meal.

If you have meal prep sorted, you will have plenty of frozen meals ready for the week that are packed with healthy ingredients and no preservatives. The best part? You can simply pop them in the air fryer and dinner is ready in no time. Keep an eye out for the recipes in the next chapters that can be prepared in advance.

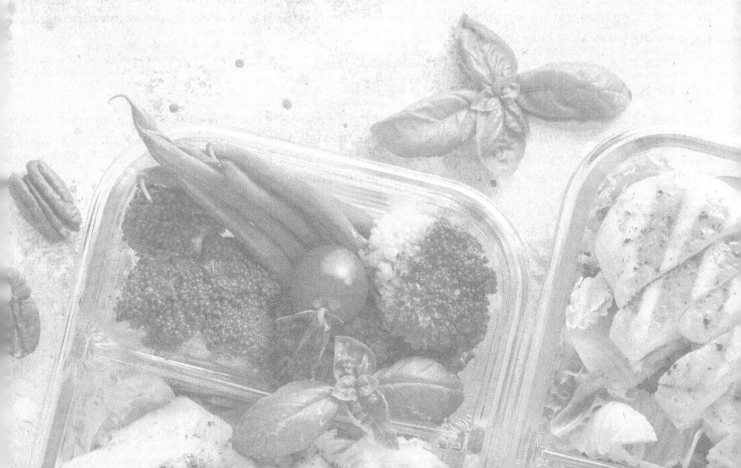

A Guide to Air Frying

While air fryers are incredibly simple to use, there are some key points to note if you are new to air frying. These include some common mistakes people make when using an air fryer, as well as the right foods to cook in the air fryer

Top Mistakes When Using an Air Fryer

These are a few common mistakes people make when using an air fryer and I would like to help you avoid these mistakes from the beginning. I have made a few of them myself and they range from wrong cooking methods to not cooking the right foods. So, if you have been using an air fryer already, you may have noticed things not going your way entirely if you have been doing any of the following:

You Don't Check Your Food Enough

Air fryers have made it incredibly easy to pop food inside, set the time, and then leave it to cook away until the timer beeps. However, many foods could do with a few checks throughout the cooking process. Foods like salmon have a very thin line between being cooked and overcooked, so you need to be checking the food consistently. Foods like French fries need to be shaken a few times throughout the cooking process to ensure an even cook.

You Only Cook Fried Foods

You may think that air fryers are limited to cooking fried foods because of the name; however, they are an incredibly versatile kitchen appliance. You can cook meats, vegetables, and even baked goods in an air fryer. Be sure not to limit yourself to what you cook there. Since you've already picked up this book, it means you are ready to try out all the possibilities.

You Overcrowd the Basket

If you are cooking for a few people, you might toss all the food in at once to get the cooking done a lot quicker. Unfortunately, air fryers do have a limited capacity and this is for very good reasons. If you have too much food in at once, the heat won't be distributed evenly and you could have a combination of burnt and undercooked food in one basket. You should rather cook your food in batches to ensure even cooking

Best and Worst Foods to Air Fry

We already know there are plenty of foods you can enjoy in an air fryer, I managed to create 250 recipes for this cookbook, after all, yet some foods are not well-suited for air fryers. This can be due to unwanted textures that the air fryer can cause, drying out of the food, messy foods, and some foods just need water to cook properly. This does not mean you can't use these foods in your meal; you can cook some elements separately.

Best Foods for an Air Fryer	Worst Foods for an Air Fryer
French fries	Any food with a wet batter on it
Potatoes	Foods that require a lot of water such as rice or pasta
Meat and poultry	Broccoli will dry out too much
Chickpeas for a crunchy snack	Olive oil may burn at the high heats
Air-fried doughnuts	Leafy greens won't cook evenly
Chicken nuggets	Salmon can overcook easily if you aren't carefully monitoring it
Small pizzas to create a crispy base	Cakes will dry out in an air fryer
Crispy zucchini	Bacon will splash too much oil and create a mess in the air fryer
Frozen foods, including fried foods, frozen veggies, and frozen prepared meals	Too much cheese can cause a mess in the air fryer if it melts all over

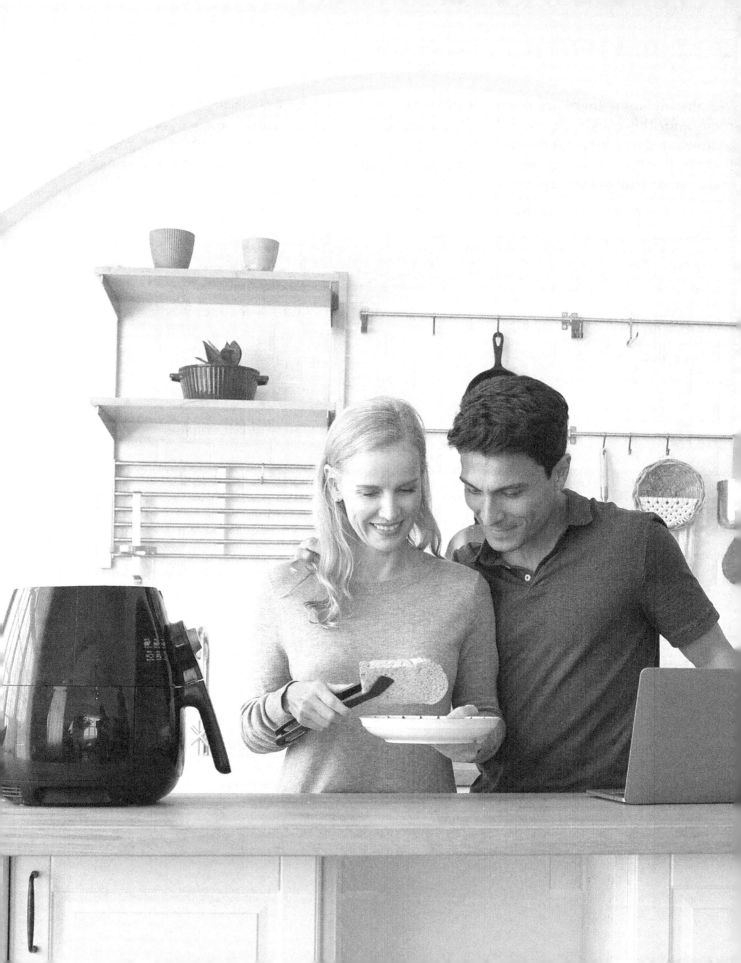

Choosing the Right Air Fryer

There are many considerations to take into account when purchasing your air fryer, including the size, capacity, and functions. Once you have considered these, you should be able to choose the right air fryer for you.

The Size

When purchasing an air fryer, you should consider the amount of space in your kitchen and where you are going to place the air fryer. Will it fit comfortably in this area with access to a plug point, and will the draw of the air fryer have enough room to open fully?

The Capacity

Next, the inside of the air fryer is important. Is there enough room to cook the amount of food you will be cooking? If you are only cooking for yourself, you may opt for a smaller model to work within your budget and to save on your energy bill. However, if you are cooking for a larger family, you should consider a bigger air fryer so you don't have to keep cooking in batches, since it will likely cost you more money on energy in the long run.

The Functions

Once you have chosen your size, are you looking for something with simple cooking functions, or would you like a more complex model that offers dehydration abilities or a toaster oven? You can also look for models with pre-programmed settings for the foods you will be cooking the most. You should also consider the temperature abilities of the air fryer. Make sure you choose a model that can heat up high enough if you will be cooking whole chickens and other meats.

Top 10 Air Fryers

Model	Capacity	Functions
Ultrean Air Fryer	4.2 Quarts	<ul><li>Multifunction Cooker to fry, grill, roast, and bake</li><li>Easy to clean: dishwasher safe basket</li><li>auto switch off timer (0-30mins) and adjustable temperature setting</li></ul>
Chefman TurboFry	2 Quarts	<ul><li>Healthy frying using at least 98% less oil than traditional fryers</li><li>Space saving compact size</li><li>Easy to clean: dishwasher safe fryer basket</li></ul>
Philips Premium TurboStar	2,75 Quarts	<ul><li>Fry. bake. grill. roast, reheat functions</li><li>Fat Removal Technology for healthy meals, fry with up to 90% less fat</li><li>Rapid Air technology with 7x faster air flow</li></ul>
Ninja Air Fryer	4 Quarts	<ul><li>4 cooking functions</li><li>75 % less fat than traditional frying methods</li><li>Easy to clean: dishwasher safe parts</li></ul>
Ninja Air Fryer Max XL	5.5 Quarts	<ul><li>7 different cooking settings, including air broil and max crisp</li><li>Air fry with up to 75 % less fat than traditional frying methods</li><li>Max Crisp technology</li></ul>

Model	Capacity	Functions
COSORI Air Fryer Max XL	5.8 Quarts	- 11 presets for popular dishes - 85% less oil than traditional deep-frying methods - Digital display
COMFEE' Digital Air Fryer	5.8 Quarts	- 8 preset functions - The hot air fryers oven can reduce 90% oil for healthy diets - User Friendly and safe to use
GoWISE GW22956-7	7 Quarts	- 8 presets for popular dishes - Touchscreen display - 3 dehydrating racks
GoWISE USA 7-Quart Electric Air Fryer	7 Quarts	- 8 different cooking functions - Can cook large batches at once - Compact and sleek design
Instant Pot Vortex Plus	10 Quarts	- 7 built-in smart programs, including: bake, roast, toast, broil, dehydrate and rotisserie - Deep-fried flavor with little to no oil for healthy meals - Easy to clean

Recipes

Breakfast - 17

Snacks & Side Dishes - 29

Beef, Pork & Lamb - 36

Poultry - 48

Fish & Seafood - 60

Plant Based - 72

Desserts - 79

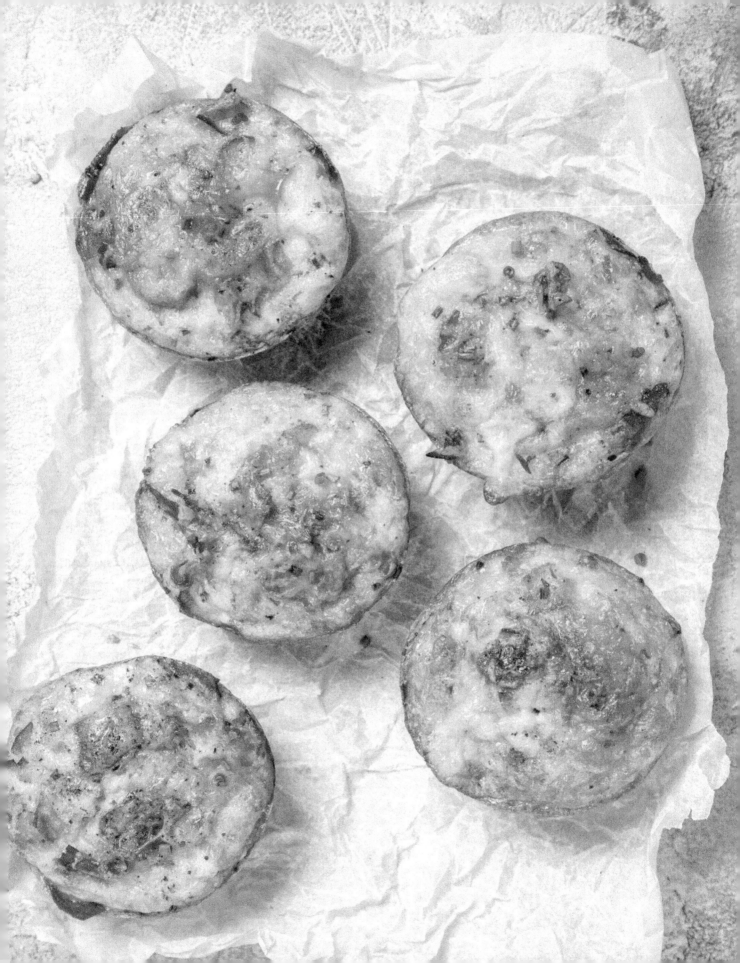

BREAKFAST

1. Air Fried Asparagus

INGREDIENTS | Servings: 2
- 3 slices avocado
- 2 bread pieces
- 3 ham, slices
- ½ tomato, slices
- 1 tbsp. oil
- 3 sticks asparagus
- 1 egg

DIRECTIONS | Ready in about: 22 min

Beat the egg in a bowl. Add the avocado, ham, and asparagus. Mix well. Take a round pan and grease the oil. Pour the mixture with a pinch of tomato slices. Put in the air fryer. Place the pieces of bread on the sides of the pan. Bake 15 minutes at 300°F. When you are ready, serve and enjoy.

2. Air Fried Sandwich

INGREDIENTS | Servings: 2
- 2 eggs
- salt and black pepper to the taste
- 2 English muffins, halved
- 2 bacon strips

DIRECTIONS | Ready in about: 16 min

Crack the eggs in your air fryer, add the bacon on top, cover, and cook at 390°F for 6 minutes. Heat the English muffin halves in the microwave for a few seconds, divide the eggs into 2 halves, add the bacon on top, season with salt and pepper, top with the 2 more English muffins, and serve for breakfast

3. Amazing Crab Breakfast

INGREDIENTS | Servings: 2
- 3 cloves garlic, minced
- 1 lb. crabmeat
- hot sauce to taste
- 1 cup Swiss cheddar
- salt and pepper to taste

DIRECTIONS | Ready in about: 14 min

Place the crab meat and garlic in a bowl. Mix with your hands and add the hot sauce, salt, and pepper.

Add the cheese and mix well. Make round meatballs and put them in the air fryer. Cook the meatballs for 10 minutes at 300°F. Once cooked, serve and enjoy.

4. Asparagus Frittata

INGREDIENTS | Servings: 2
- 2 tbsp. parmesan, grated
- 4 eggs, whisked
- 10 asparagus tips, steamed
- 4 tbsp. milk
- cooking spray
- Salt and black pepper to taste

DIRECTIONS | Ready in about: 15 min

In a portable bowl, combine the eggs with the Parmesan, milk, salt, and pepper and beat well. Warmth the air fryer to 400°F and grease with cooking spray. Add the asparagus, add the mixed eggs, mix a little and cook for 5 minutes. Divide the omelet between plates and serve for breakfast.

5. Bacon and Ham Mix

INGREDIENTS | Servings: 2
- 6 bread slices
- 1 cup ham, chopped
- salt to taste
- 3 eggs
- 4 bacon, slices
- 1 cup Cheddar cheese
- ½ cup milk

DIRECTIONS | Ready in about: 15 min

Beat the eggs in a bowl. Add the ham, cheese, milk, and salt. Mix well and add the bacon slices. Grab a round baking sheet and pour the mixture into it. Bake for 10 minutes in an air fryer at 300°F. When finished, serve with slices of bread and enjoy your meal.

6. Bell Pepper Breakfast Mix

INGREDIENTS | **Servings:** 2
- 1 chopped green bell pepper
- 1 onion – chopped
- 5 chopped mushrooms
- salt and pepper to taste
- 2 eggs

DIRECTIONS | **Ready in about:** 22 min

Peel the beets and cut them into chips. Then place the beet slices in the air fryer in a layer and sprinkle with olive oil. Bake the beetroot fries for 14 minutes at 365°F. When the time is up and the fries are done, give it time to cool and serve.

7. Black Beans with Eggs

INGREDIENTS | **Servings:** 2
- 4 eggs
- 2 tbsp. olive oil
- salt and pepper to taste
- 1 cup black beans
- 3 tbsp. salsa (anyone you like)
- 1 avocado, sliced

DIRECTIONS | **Ready in about:** 20 min

Beat the eggs in a bowl. Add the avocado, salsa, black beans, salt, and pepper. Spurt the mixture into the round pan and grease it with oil. Leave to cook in the air fryer for 14 minutes at 300°F. When finished, serve and enjoy!

8. Broccoli Breakfast Mix

INGREDIENTS | **Servings:** 2
- 2 tbsp. mayonnaise
- 1 tbsp. butter
- ½ cup mushroom soup
- 1 onion, sliced
- 1 cup broccoli, chopped
- salt and pepper to taste
- ½ lb. chicken, cooked and mashed

DIRECTIONS | **Ready in about:** 20 min

Add the chicken to the bowl. Combine mayonnaise, mushroom soup, onion, broccoli, and salt and pepper. Grease the round pan with the butter. Add the mixture to the pan. Bake in an air fryer for 14 minutes at 300°F. When finished, serve and enjoy.

9. Broccoli Quiche

INGREDIENTS | **Servings:** 2
- 1 tomato, chopped
- 1 broccoli head, florets separated and steamed
- 3 carrots, chopped and steamed
- 2 eggs
- 2 ounces cheddar cheese, grated
- 2 ounces milk
- salt and black pepper to taste
- 1 tsp. thyme, chopped
- 1 tsp. parsley, chopped

DIRECTIONS | **Ready in about:** 30 min

In a portable bowl, combine the eggs with the milk, parsley, thyme, salt, and pepper and beat well. Put the broccoli, carrots, and tomato in your air fryer. Add the mixed eggs on top, sprinkle with cheddar cheese, cover, and bake at 350°F for 20 minutes. Divide among plates and serve for breakfast.

10. Carrot Mixed Chicken

INGREDIENTS | Servings: 2
- 2 tomatoes, chopped
- cilantro to garnish
- 1 lb. chicken breast, chopped
- 1 carrot, chopped
- ½ tsp. red chili powder
- 2 minced garlic cloves
- 1 cup cheese, shredded

DIRECTIONS | Ready in about: 20 min

Add the chicken to a portable bowl with the tomatoes. Mix well. Add the carrot, garlic, red pepper powder, and cheese. Mix well. Make meatballs with the mixture and put them in the air fryer. Cook for 15 minutes at 300°F. Once cooked, garnish with cilantro and serve!

11. Cheese Burger Patties

INGREDIENTS | Servings: 2
- salt and pepper to taste
- 4 cheeseburger patties
- 1 tbsp. steak sauce
- 1 cup Cheddar cheese
- ½ small pack of French fries (frozen)
- 4 hamburger buns

DIRECTIONS | Ready in about: 25 min

Place the burgers in the air fryer. Add cheese, meat sauce with salt and pepper. Add the fries around an empty space in the air fryer. Cook in your air fryer for 20 minutes at 300°F. Once cooked, place each burger on the bread and enjoy with the fries.

12. Chicken Mix

INGREDIENTS | Servings: 2
- ½ cup buttermilk
- 1 lb. boneless chicken, chopped
- 1 tbsp. Cayenne pepper
- 1 cup flour (all-purpose)
- salt to taste

For Maple Sauce:
- 2 tbsp. maple syrup
- salt to taste
- 2 tbsp. mustard
- ½ tbsp. vegetable oil

DIRECTIONS | Ready in about: 20 min

Mix the buttermilk with the cayenne pepper in a bowl. Add salt and flour. Mix well. Spot the chicken in the pan and pour the mixture over it. Cook in an air fryer 10 minutes at 300°F. Meanwhile, prepare the sauce: In a bowl, mix the mustard, the oil plant, salt, and maple syrup. Mix well. Once cooked, remove and serve with the delicious sauce.

13. Chicken with Cheese

INGREDIENTS | Servings: 2
- parsley as needed
- 1 lb. chicken, chopped
- 2 minced garlic cloves
- salt and pepper to taste
- 4 buns
- 1 tbsp. oil
- ½ cup basil, chopped
- 1 cup breadcrumbs
- 1 cup Parmesan cheese

DIRECTIONS | Ready in about: 20 min

Add the chicken to the bowl. Combine the garlic, cheese, salt, and pepper with the basil and parsley. Grease the grill of the air fryer. Make cupcakes with the mixture and cover them with breadcrumbs. Put them in the air fryer to cook for 15 minutes at 300°F. Once cooked, serve them by placing each burger on the bread and enjoy your meal.

14. Chicken with Orange Taste

INGREDIENTS | Servings: 2
- 2 carrots, sliced
- 1 lb. chicken – boneless, shredded
- 2 onion, sliced
- ¼ cup orange juice
- Cajun seasoning
- 1 cup peas (frozen)
- parsley for garnishing
- 2 tbsp. dill

DIRECTIONS | Ready in about: 20 min

Add the chicken to the bowl. Combine the carrots, onion, orange juice, peas, and dill. Mix well. Add the mixture to the round pan. Bake for 15 minutes in an air fryer at 300°F. When finished, garnish with Cajun and parsley for serving.

15. Dates and Millet Pudding

INGREDIENTS | Servings: 2

- 7 ounces of water
- 14 ounces milk
- ⅔ cup millet
- Honey for serving
- 4 dates, pitted

DIRECTIONS | Ready in about: 25 min

Place the millet in a pan suitable for your air fryer, add the dates, milk, and water, mix, stir in your air fryer and cook at 360°F for 15 minutes. Divide among plates, sprinkle with honey and serve.

16. Delicious Shrimp

INGREDIENTS | Servings: 2

- 1 tomato, chopped
- 1 cup lettuce, chopped
- 1 lb. shrimp/prawn, chopped
- 1 tbsp. dill
- 1 cup white cabbage
- 2 tbsp. lime juice
- Cajun seasoning
- ½ cup coriander, chopped

DIRECTIONS | Ready in about: 14 min

Take a bowl and add the shrimp/prawns. Stir in the tomato, white cabbage, dill, lime juice and cilantro. Pour the mixture into a baking dish. Cook for 10 minutes in an air fryer at 350°F. When it is ready, sprinkle with lettuce and Cajun. Serve and enjoy delicious food.

17. Delicious Tofu and Mushrooms

INGREDIENTS | Servings: 2

- 1 cup panko breadcrumbs
- 1 tofu block, pressed and cut into medium pieces
- 1 tbsp. mushrooms, minced
- salt and black pepper to taste
- 1 egg
- ½ tbsp. flour

DIRECTIONS | Ready in about: 20 min

In a bowl, combine the egg with the mushrooms, flour, salt, and pepper and beat well. Plunge the tofu pieces in the egg mixture, then slide them into the panko breadcrumbs, place the mixture in your air fryer, and cook at 350°F for 10 minutes. Serve them immediately for breakfast.

18. Dill Eggs

INGREDIENTS | Servings: 2

- 2 minced garlic cloves
- 1 tbsp. dill
- 1 tbsp. vinegar
- salt and pepper to taste
- 1 tbsp. oil
- 1 tbsp. oregano
- 1 tomato, sliced
- 1 cup olives
- 1 onion, chopped
- 3 eggs

DIRECTIONS | Ready in about: 22 min

Beat the eggs in a bowl. Add the garlic, dill, vinegar, oregano, tomato, olives, and onion. Grease the round pan with oil. Pour the mixture into the pan. Bake in the air fryer for 18 minutes at 300°F. When done, serve!

19. Egg Sauce Breakfast

INGREDIENTS | Servings: 2

- 1 tbsp. butter
- 2 muffins
- 2 cups spinach, chopped
- 1 tsp. vinegar
- 2 eggs

For the Sauce:

- 1 tbsp. Lemon juice
- 2 egg yolk
- 2 pinch salt and pepper
- 1 tbsp. butter
- ½ cup water

DIRECTIONS | Ready in about: 20 min

Beat the eggs in a bowl. Add the vinegar, spinach, and butter. Mix well. Place the muffins in the pan and pour the mixture. Cook in an air fryer for 15 minutes at 300°F. Make the sauce: Combine the egg yolk, lemon juice, water, butter, salt, and pepper. Beat until light and fluffy. When the cooking is done, take it out and serve it with the sauce!

20. Eggs with Onion

INGREDIENTS | Servings: 2
- 1 tbsp. mustard
- 1 tbsp. mayonnaise
- 1 onion, chopped
- 1 tbsp. paprika
- ½ tsp. vinegar
- salt and pepper to taste
- 2 eggs

DIRECTIONS | Ready in about: 15 min

Beat the eggs in a bowl. Add the mayonnaise, mustard, and vinegar. After mixing well, add the onion, paprika, and salt. Pour the mixture into the round pan. Cook 10 minutes in the air fryer at 300°F. Once cooked, serve and enjoy.

21. Fish and Bread

INGREDIENTS | Servings: 2
- salt and pepper to taste
- 4 bread, slices
- 1 small fish, canned
- 2 tbsp. mayonnaise

DIRECTIONS | Ready in about: 15 min

Add the fish to a bowl with the mayonnaise. Add salt and pepper. Mix well. Add the mixture to a round pan. Put it in the air fryer for 10 minutes at 300°F. Place the pieces of bread on the side of the pan. When you're done, serve!

22. Fluffy Egg

INGREDIENTS | Servings: 2
- 1 cup pumpkin puree
- 1½ cup milk
- 2 egg
- 2 tbsp. vinegar
- 2 tbsp. oil
- 2 cups flour (all-purpose)
- 1 tsp. baking soda
- 2 tsp. baking powder
- 1 tbsp. brown sugar
- 1 tsp. cinnamon powder

DIRECTIONS | Ready in about: 16 min

Beat the eggs in a bowl. Add milk, pumpkin puree, flour, baking powder, baking soda, brown sugar, and ground cinnamon. Mix well and add the milk. Grease the pan with oil and spurt the mixture. Put it in the air fryer for 10 minutes at 300°F. When it's done, enjoy!

23. French Toast Delight

INGREDIENTS | Servings: 2
- 2 tbsp. butter
- 4 bread slices
- ½ tsp. cinnamon
- pinch nutmeg icing sugar and maple syrup, to serve
- pinch of salt
- 2 eggs
- pinch of ground cloves

DIRECTIONS | Ready in about: 20 min

Preheat the air fryer to 350°F. Whisk together the eggs, cloves, cinnamon, nutmeg, cloves, and salt in a bowl. Butter the sides of each slice of bread and cut them into strips. Dip the buttered bread slices one after the other in the egg mixture and place them in the pan. Cook for 2 minutes, then remove the strips. Lightly coat bread strips with cooking spray on both sides. Spot the pan in the air fryer and cook for another 4 minutes, making sure they cook evenly. Remove the bread from the air fryer once it is golden brown. Sprinkle with powdered sugar and drizzle with maple syrup.

24. Garlic and Cheese Bread Rolls

INGREDIENTS | Servings: 2
- 6 tsp. of melted butter
- 2 bread rolls
- 8 tbsp. of grated cheese
- garlic bread spice mix

DIRECTIONS | Ready in about: 12 min

Cut sandwiches from the top across, but do not cut them from the bottom. Place all the cheese in the slits and brush the tops of the sandwiches with melted butter. Sprinkle the garlic mixture over the muffins. Heat the air fryer to 350°F. Place the rolls in the basket and cook until the cheese has melted, about 5 minutes.

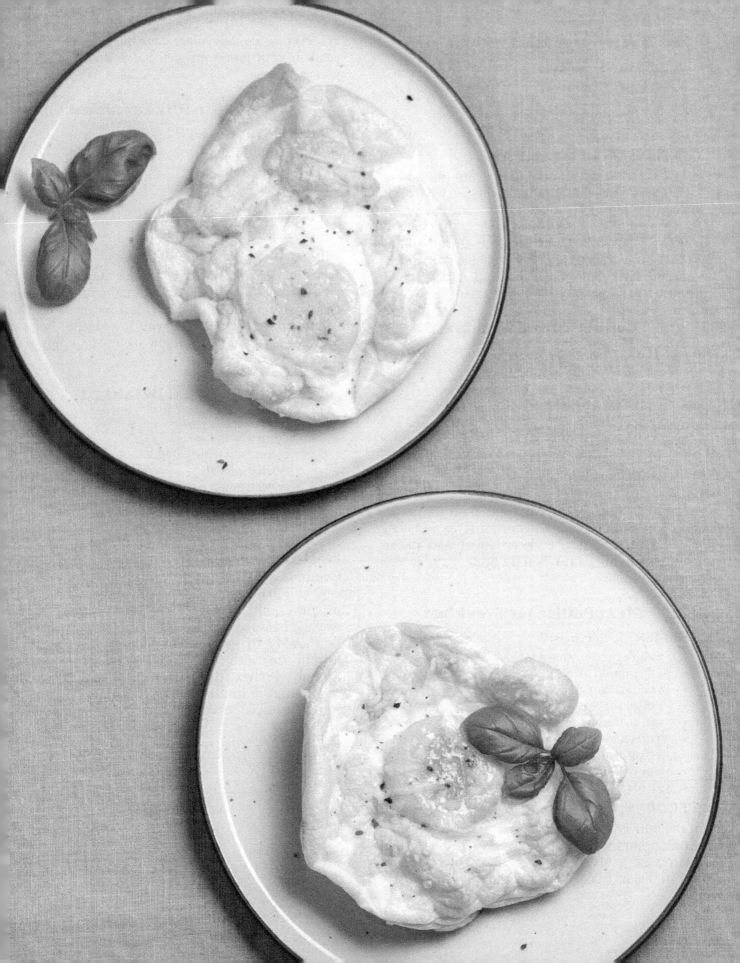

25. Hearty Breakfast with Bacon

INGREDIENTS | **Servings:** 2
- 4 strips of bacon
- 4 eggs
- 4 slices of toast
- salt and pepper to taste

DIRECTIONS | **Ready in about:** 20 min

Flatten the toast with a rolling pin. Cut out a large round area and divide it in the center. Fry bacon in the air fryer at 300°F for 5 minutes. Line the muffin cups with 2 half circles of toast each so that there is no space. Then, fill each with bacon and season an egg. Season with pepper and salt. Place the muffins in the air fryer basket and bake at 350°F for 10 minutes.

26. Lettuce Mixed Breakfast

INGREDIENTS | **Servings:** 2
- 2 tbsp. ranch dressing
- 1 tbsp. hot sauce
- 1 lb. chicken breast, chopped
- 1 cup Mozzarella cheese, shredded
- 1 cup lettuce leaves
- 4 bread pieces

DIRECTIONS | **Ready in about:** 11 min

Combine chicken and ranch dressing in a bowl. Add the hot sauce and cheese. Mix well. Pour it into the round pan. Spot the pan in your air fryer and cook for 5 minutes at 300°F. Keep the bread pieces separate from the pan. When it's done, serve it with some lettuce leaves!

27. Meat Patties for Breakfast

INGREDIENTS | **Servings:** 2
- 3 cloves garlic, minced
- 1 lb. ground meat
- 1 onion, chopped
- 1 tbsp. garlic powder
- 1 tbsp. Cumin powder
- 2 green onions, chopped
- 2 tbsp. tomato sauce
- 4 burger buns
- 1 cup cheese, shredded

DIRECTIONS | **Ready in about:** 15 min

Put the minced meat with garlic in a bowl. Now mix the onion, cumin powder, garlic powder, cheese, and tomato sauce. Mix well. Make meatballs and put them in the air fryer. Cook for 10 minutes at 300°F. When you are ready, place each burger on bread and garnish with green onions. Serve and enjoy when you're ready!

28. Muffin Mix Breakfast

INGREDIENTS | **Servings:** 2
- 1 tbsp. oil
- 1 egg
- 1 muffin whole wheat
- black pepper to taste
- 1 cup of cheese, shredded
- 4 slices of Canadian bacon

DIRECTIONS | **Ready in about:** 20 min

Beat the egg in a bowl. Add black pepper and mix well. Grease the round pan with oil and pour in the egg mixture. Add the cheese and bacon. Place the round pan in the air fryer with the muffin. Bake 12 minutes at 300°F. When you are ready, enjoy your meal!

29. Oatmeal Breakfast

INGREDIENTS | **Servings:** 2
- 2 eggs
- 3 ounces butter melted ½ cup flour
- 3½ ounces oats
- ¼ tsp. vanilla essence
- 1 tbsp. raisins Cooking spray
- ½ cup icing sugar
- 1 pinch baking powder

DIRECTIONS | **Ready in about:** 20 min

Combine sugar and butter until smooth. Beat the eggs and the vanilla extract. Add to the sugar/butter mixture until soft peaks form. Combine flour, raisins, baking powder, and oatmeal in a separate bowl. Add it to the mixed ingredients. Lightly grease muffin cups with cooking spray and fill with batter mixture. Preheat the air fryer to 350°F. Place the mold muffin in the air fryer pan. Cook for 12 minutes. Relax, serve, and savor!

30. Potato Mix Breakfast

INGREDIENTS | **Servings:** 2

- 1 lb. steak, sliced
- 2 cups Provolone cheese
- 1 onion, chopped
- 1 tbsp. butter
- 1 potato, diced
- salt and pepper to taste
- 4 bread, slices
- 1 tbsp. oil

DIRECTIONS | **Ready in about:** 15 min

Add cheese and potatoes to a bowl. Combine the onion, butter, salt, and pepper. Mix well. Grease the round pan with oil and pour the mixture, placing the steak on the mixture. Bake 10 minutes at 300°F. Once cooked, serve with slices of bread and enjoy your meal.

31. Quick Eggs

INGREDIENTS | **Servings:** 2

- 4 slices bread
- salt and pepper to taste
- 2 eggs
- 2 tbsp. butter

DIRECTIONS | **Ready in about:** 15 min

Beat the eggs in a bowl. Add the butter. Mix well. Add salt and pepper. Pour the mixture into the round pan. Bake at 300°F for 10 minutes, setting aside the bread pieces. When you're done, enjoy a quick and easy breakfast!

32. Rarebit Air Fried Egg

INGREDIENTS | **Servings:** 2

- 4 eggs
- 4 slices sourdough
- ⅓ cup ale
- 1 tsp. mustard powder
- 1½ cups cheddar, grated
- ½ tsp. paprika
- 2 tsp. Worcestershire sauce
- black pepper to taste

DIRECTIONS | **Ready in about:** 10 min

Fry the eggs with the sunny side up and set aside. Preheat the air fryer to 350°F. In a bowl, combine the cheddar cheese, beer, paprika, mustard powder, and Worcestershire sauce. Unfurl only one side of each slice of sourdough with the cheddar cheese mixture. Place the slices of bread in the air fryer tray. Cook for approximate 3 minutes until lightly browned. Top the slices of bread with fried eggs and season with pepper to taste.

33. Salmon Breakfast with Carrot Mix

INGREDIENTS | **Servings:** 2

- 1 lb. salmon, chopped
- 4 bread slices
- 1 carrot, shredded
- 3 tbsp. pickled red onion
- 2 cups feta crumbled
- 2 cucumber, slices

DIRECTIONS | **Ready in about:** 21 min

Put the salmon with the feta cheese in a bowl. Add the carrot, cucumber, and red onion. Mix well. Make a layer of bread on the baking sheet, then pour the mixture over it. Leave to cook in the fryer for 15 minutes at 300°F. Once cooked, serve and enjoy.

34. Salmon Mixed Eggs

INGREDIENTS | **Servings:** 2

- 2 eggs
- 1 lb. salmon, cooked
- 1 onion, chopped
- salt and pepper to taste
- 1 tbsp. oil
- 1 cup celery, chopped

DIRECTIONS | **Ready in about:** 16 min

Beat the eggs in a bowl. Add the celery, onion, salt, and pepper. Add the oil to the round pan and pour the mixture. Put it in the air fryer at 300°F. Let it cook for 10 minutes. Once cooked, serve and enjoy with the cooked salmon.

35. Scrambled Eggs

INGREDIENTS | **Servings:** 2
- 2 tbsp. butter
- 2 eggs
- salt and black pepper to taste
- pinch of sweet paprika
- 1 red bell pepper, chopped

DIRECTIONS | **Ready in about:** 20 min

In a portable bowl, combine the eggs with the salt, pepper, paprika, and red pepper and beat well. Heat the air fryer to 140°F, add the butter, and let it melt. Add the mixed eggs, mix, and cook for 10 minutes. Divide the scrambled eggs among plates and serve for breakfast.

36. Shallot Mix

INGREDIENTS | **Servings:** 2
- 1 small shallot
- 2 minced garlic cloves
- 1 tbsp. vegetable oil
- ½ cup cream
- 1 cup cheddar cheese
- salt and pepper to taste
- 1 cup lettuce, chopped
- ½ cup mint, minced
- ½ cup olives
- 1 cup zucchini, chopped

DIRECTIONS | **Ready in about:** 20 min

Take a bowl and add the shallot and garlic. Combine the cheese, cream, salt and pepper, olives, and mint. Mix well. Take the round pan. Grease with oil. Include the mixture to the pan and spread over the chopped zucchini. Bake in the air fryer for 19 minutes at 300°F.

37. Simple Bacon and Eggs

INGREDIENTS | **Servings:** 2
- 3 egg whites
- 3 eggs
- ½ cup milk
- ½ tbsp. green pepper
- 3 dices mushrooms
- 4 bread pieces
- 3 cheese, slices
- 2 slices bacon

DIRECTIONS | **Ready in about:** 15 min

Beat the eggs and the white in a bowl. Add the milk, mushrooms, green pepper, and bacon. Mix well. Pour the mixture into a round pan and add the cheese. Place the bread slices on the sides of the test in the air fryer. Bake 10 minutes at 300°F. When you're ready, serve and enjoy!

38. Simple Bacon

INGREDIENTS | **Servings:** 2
- ½ tsp. paprika
- 8 strips bacon
- salt and pepper to taste
- ½ cup cheddar cheese
- 1 tbsp. Cayenne powder
- 1 tbsp. garlic powder
- 4 hamburger patties
- 1 tomato, chopped
- 4 hamburger buns

DIRECTIONS | **Ready in about:** 25 min

Take the round pan and place the patties as the bottom layer. Add the paprika, salt and pepper, garlic powder, tomato, and cayenne pepper, and garnish with cheese. Cook in your air fryer for 20 minutes at 300°F. Also, heat the sandwiches in the air fryer for 2 minutes. Once cooked, put the meatballs on the sandwich and serve.

39. Simple Breakfast

INGREDIENTS | **Servings:** 2
- 1 lb. steak
- ½ cup cheese, shredded
- 1 bell pepper, sliced
- 1 onion, sliced

DIRECTIONS | **Ready in about:** 14 min

Place the steak on the baking sheet. Put the slices of pepper and onion. Spread the cheese. Cook in your air fryer for 10 minutes at 300°F. Once cooked, serve and enjoy.

40. Smoked Air Fried Tofu

INGREDIENTS | **Servings:** 2
- salt and black pepper to taste
- 1 tofu block, pressed and cubed
- 1 tbsp. smoked paprika
- cooking spray
- ¼ cup cornstarch

DIRECTIONS | **Ready in about:** 22 min

Grease the basket of your air fryer with cooking spray and heat the fryer to 370°F. In a bowl, combine the tofu with salt, pepper, smoked paprika, and cornstarch and mix well. Add the tofu to your air fryer basket and cook for 12 minutes, shaking the fryer every 4 minutes. Divide into bowls and serve for breakfast.

41. Spinach Breakfast Parcels

INGREDIENTS | **Servings:** 2
- 1 pound baby spinach leaves, roughly chopped
- 4 sheets filo pastry
- ½ pound ricotta cheese
- 1 egg, whisked
- 2 tbsp. pine nuts
- zest from 1 lemon, grated
- salt and black pepper to taste
- Greek yogurt for serving

DIRECTIONS | **Ready in about:** 15 min

In a portable bowl, combine the spinach with the cheese, egg, lemon zest, salt, pepper, and pine nuts and mix. Place the twine leaves on a work surface, divide the spinach mixture, fold them diagonally to form the bunches, and place them in your preheated air fryer at 400°F. Cook the bunches for 4 minutes, divide them into plates and serve with Greek yogurt on the side.

42. Spinach Mushroom Mix

INGREDIENTS | **Servings:** 2
- 1 onion, chopped
- 1 tbsp. oil
- 6 small mushrooms, chopped
- 1 cup spinach
- 2 minced garlic cloves
- ½ cup parsley, chopped
- salt and pepper to taste
- 2 cups of milk
- almonds for seasoning
- 3 cups chicken, shredded

DIRECTIONS | **Ready in about:** 15 min

Place the chicken in a bowl. Combine the onion, mushrooms, garlic, spinach, and parsley. Mix well. Add the milk, salt, and pepper. Get a round baking pan. Grease with oil. Add the mixture. Cook in your air fryer for 10 minutes at 300°F. Once cooked, serve with almond vinaigrette.

43. Steak Strips

INGREDIENTS | **Servings:** 2
- salt and pepper to taste
- 5 strips steak
- 6 slices Ciabatta bread
- 1 tomato, chopped
- ½ cup cheese, shredded
- 2 tbsp. garlic, chopped
- ½ cup basil, chopped

DIRECTIONS | **Ready in about:** 20 min

Mix the cheese with the basil in a bowl. Add the garlic and tomato with salt and pepper. Spurt the mixture into the round pan and arrange the fillets in strips. Leave to cook in the air fryer at 300°F for 15 minutes. When you are done, serve them with bread and enjoy your meal.

44. Thai Style Omelette

INGREDIENTS | **Servings:** 2

- 2 eggs
- 1 tbsp. fish salt
- 3½ ounces minced pork
- 1 cup onion, chopped

DIRECTIONS | **Ready in about:** 15 min

Beat the eggs until light and fluffy. Preheat the air fryer to air at 280°F. Add all ingredients to a bowl. Pour the mixture into the pan of the air fryer. Remove after 10 minutes or when the tortilla is golden brown. Cut and serve.

45. Tofu for Breakfast

INGREDIENTS | **Servings:** 2

- 1 tbsp. oil
- 1 tbsp. peppercorns
- salt and pepper to taste
- 1 tbsp. coriander seeds
- 4 buns
- 1 tbsp. paprika
- 2 cups tofu
- 1 bay leaf
- 1 onion, sliced
- ½ cup lettuce, shredded

DIRECTIONS | **Ready in about:** 24 min

Grease the round pan with oil. Add the tofu, salt and pepper, cilantro seeds, paprika, bay leaf and onion to a bowl. Mix well. Pour into the pan. Bake in the air fryer for 20 minutes at 300°F. When done, top with lettuce and serve with sandwiches.

46. Turkey Burrito

INGREDIENTS | **Servings:** 2

- ½ red bell pepper, sliced
- 4 slices of turkey breast already cooked
- 2 eggs
- 2 tbsp. salsa
- 1 small avocado, peeled, pitted, and sliced
- salt and black pepper to taste
- tortillas for serving
- ⅛ cup mozzarella cheese, grated

DIRECTIONS | **Ready in about:** 20 min

In a portable bowl, beat the eggs with salt and pepper to taste, pour them into a pan and place them in the basket of the fryer. Bake at 400°F for 5 minutes, remove the pan from the fryer and transfer the eggs to a plate. Arrange the tortillas on a work surface, distribute the eggs on top, distribute the turkey meat, pepper, cheese, sauce, and avocado evenly. Roll up your burritos and place them in the air fryer after covering them with foil. Heat the burritos to 300°F for 3 minutes, divide into plates and serve.

47. Veggie Mix

INGREDIENTS | **Servings:** 2

- chopped Spinach
- ½ cup milk
- 1 cup cheese, shredded
- ½ bell pepper, chopped
- ½ onion, chopped
- 1 tbsp. oil
- 4 eggs
- ½ cup mint, chopped
- salt and pepper to taste

DIRECTIONS | **Ready in about:** 20 min

Beat the eggs in a bowl. Add the milk, cheese, spinach, onion, bell pepper, salt and pepper, and mint. Take the round pan. Grease with oil. Pour the mixture into the pan. Leave to cook in the air fryer for 14 minutes at 300°F. When finished, serve and enjoy!

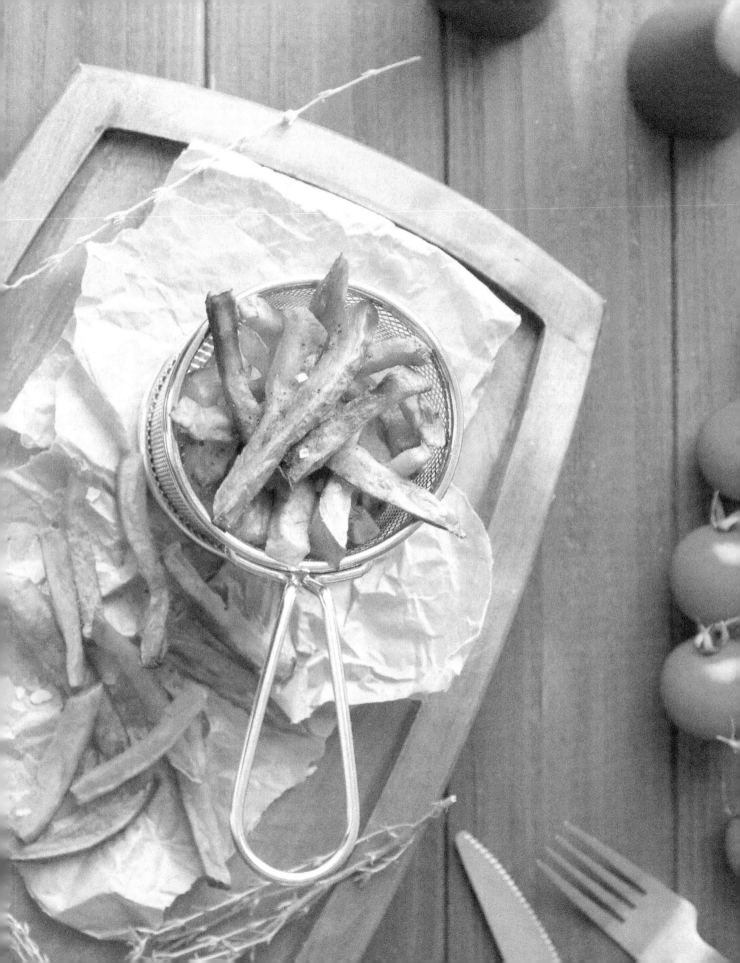

SNACKS & SIDE DISHES

48. Air Fried Cheeseburger

INGREDIENTS | **Servings:** 2
- 2 bread rolls
- 2 slices of Cheddar Cheese
- ½ pound of ground beef
- 2 tsp. of salt
- 2 tbsp. of melted butter
- ½ tsp. of black pepper, ground

DIRECTIONS | **Ready in about:** 15 min

Heat the air fryer to 390°F. Shaping ground beef to form 2 meatballs. Sprinkle with salt and pepper. Cut the sandwiches in the center and place each burger in them. Place the burgers in the cooking basket and cook for about 11 minutes. Add the cheddar cheese to the meatballs and cook 1 minute longer until the cheese is melted.

49. Avocado Fries

INGREDIENTS | **Servings:** 2
- salt and black pepper to taste
- 1 avocado, pitted, peeled, sliced and cut into medium fries
- 1 tbsp. olive oil
- ½ cup panko breadcrumbs
- 1 egg, whisked
- 1 tbsp. lemon juice

DIRECTIONS | **Ready in about:** 15 min

In a bowl, combine the panko with salt and pepper and toss. In another bowl, combine the egg with a pinch of salt and beat. In a third bowl, combine the avocado fries with lemon juice and oil and mix. Dip fried in egg, then panko, place them in the basket of the air fryer and cook at 390°F for 10 minutes, shaking halfway. Divide between plates and serve as a garnish.

50. Avocado Sticks

INGREDIENTS | **Servings:** 2
- ¼ tsp. thyme
- 1 avocado, stoned
- ½ tsp. turmeric
- 1 tbsp. coconut flour
- 1 egg
- ¾ tsp. salt

DIRECTIONS | **Ready in about:** 20 min

Rind the avocado and cut it into sticks. Then sprinkle the avocado sticks with thyme, turmeric and salt. Crack the egg and beat. Place the avocado sticks in the egg mixture and cover well. Then sprinkle the avocado sticks with the coconut flour and place them in the air fryer. Bake the avocado sticks for 10 minutes at 390°F, turning them halfway through cooking.

51. Cauliflower Rice

INGREDIENTS | **Servings:** 2
- 1 tbsp. sesame oil
- 1 tbsp. peanut oil
- 4 tbsp. soy sauce
- 1 tbsp. ginger, grated
- 3 garlic cloves, minced
- juice from ½ lemon
- 9 ounces water chestnuts, drained
- 1 cauliflower head, riced
- ¾ cup peas
- 1 egg, whisked
- 15 ounces mushrooms, chopped

DIRECTIONS | **Ready in about:** 50 min

In your air fryer, combine rice with cauliflower with peanut oil, sesame oil, the sauce soya, garlic, ginger and lemon juice, stir, cover and bake at 350°F for 20 minutes. Add the chestnuts, peas, mushrooms and egg, stir and cook at 360°F for another 20 minutes. Divide among plates and serve for breakfast.

52. Chia Seeds Snack

INGREDIENTS | **Servings:** 2
- 1 cup cream cheese
- 1 banana
- 1 cup coconut, shredded
- 3 tbsp. chia seeds

DIRECTIONS | **Ready in about:** 10 min

Add the cream cheese and coconut to the round pan. Mix the chia seeds with the banana. Put in the air fryer. Bake at 300°F for 5 minutes. When you're ready, serve!

53. Chicken Legs

INGREDIENTS | **Servings:** 2
- 1 tbsp. soy sauce
- 1 tbsp. honey
- 2 garlic cloves, minced
- 1 tbsp. ginger, chopped
- 1 lb. chicken legs
- green onion, chopped, to garnish

DIRECTIONS | **Ready in about:** 20 min

Add honey and soy sauce into the air fryer pot. Stir in the garlic, ginger, green onion and chicken thighs. Bake at 300°F for 15 minutes. When it's ready, help yourself and enjoy!

54. Chickpeas Snack

INGREDIENTS | **Servings:** 2
- 1 tbsp. oil
- 1 small can chickpeas
- salt to taste
- 1 tbsp. curry powder
- 1 tbsp. cumin powder
- 1 tbsp. sweet paprika

DIRECTIONS | **Ready in about:** 12 min

Add oil into the air fryer pot. Combine the chickpeas, sweet paprika, salt, cumin powder and curry powder. Bake at 400°F for 10 minutes. When it's ready, serve it and enjoy the crispy chickpeas.

55. Coconut Cream Potatoes

INGREDIENTS | **Servings:** 2
- salt and black pepper to taste
- 1 egg, whisked
- ½ tbsp. cheddar cheese, grated
- 2 ounces coconut cream
- 1 potatoe, sliced
- ½ tbsp. flour

DIRECTIONS | **Ready in about:** 30 min

Spot the potato slices in the air fryer basket and cook at 360°F for 10 minutes. Meanwhile, in a bowl, combine the egg with the coconut cream, salt, pepper and flour. Place the potato slices in a frying pan, add the coconut cream on top, sprinkle with cheese, return to the fryer basket and bake at 400°F for 10 minutes more. Divide between plates and serve as a garnish.

56. Corn Tortilla Chips

INGREDIENTS | **Servings:** 2
- 8 corn tortillas
- salt to taste
- 6 tsp. of vegetable oil

DIRECTIONS | **Ready in about:** 8 min

Heat the air fryer to 390°F. Cut out the shapes tortillas with a utility knife. Grease tortillas with oil using a pastry brush. Place half of the tortilla in the air fryer basket and cook for 3 minutes. Repeat a similar cycle with the subsequent batch until all the fries are done. Add salt and serve hot with the sauce.

57. Corn with Lime and Cheese

INGREDIENTS | **Servings:** 2
- 1 drizzle of olive oil
- 2 corns on the cob, husks removed
- ½ cup feta cheese, grated
- juice from 2 limes
- 2 tsp. sweet paprika

DIRECTIONS | **Ready in about:** 25 min

Rub the corn with oil and paprika, put it in the air fryer, and bake at 400°F for 15 minutes, turning it once. Divide the corn between plates, sprinkle with cheese, drizzle with lemon juice, and serve as a garnish. Enjoy!

58. Corncobs

INGREDIENTS | **Servings:** 2
- 6 corncobs
- 1 cup flour
- 3 cup chives
- 1 cup milk
- 3 eggs
- 1 lb. crabmeat, minced
- 2 tbsp. oil

DIRECTIONS | **Ready in about:** 18 min

Add oil into the air fryer pot. Combine the flour, milk, eggs, corn on the cob, crab meat and chives. Bake at 350°F for 15 minutes.

59. Cornmeal Mix Snack

INGREDIENTS | **Servings:** 2
- 2 tbsp. oil
- 2 tbsp. cornmeal
- 1 cup flour
- 3 cup corn kernels
- 3 cup cheddar cheese
- 1 red chili, chopped
- 3 cup buttermilk
- 1 egg
- butter to soften, if needed

DIRECTIONS | **Ready in about:** 14 min

Add oil into the air fryer pot. Mix the cornmeal, flour, corn kernels, red pepper, buttermilk and egg. Pour into the pot. Bake at 300°F for 10 minutes. When ready, top with cheese and serve.

60. Creamy Air Fried Potato

INGREDIENTS | **Servings:** 2
- 2 bacon strips, cooked and chopped
- 1 big potato
- 1 tsp. olive oil
- 1 tbsp. green onions, chopped
- ⅓ cup cheddar cheese, shredded
- salt and black pepper to taste
- 2 tbsp. heavy cream
- 1 tbsp. butter

DIRECTIONS | **Ready in about:** 1 h 30 min

Rub the potato with oil, season with salt and pepper, put it in a preheated air fryer and bake at 400°F for 30 minutes. Turn the potato over, cook for another 30 minutes, transfer to a cutting board, let cool, cut in half lengthwise and collect the pulp in a bowl. Add the bacon, cheese, butter, cream, chives, salt and pepper, mix well and fill the potato skins with this mixture. Return the potatoes to your air fryer and bake them at 400°F for 20 minutes. Divide between plates and serve as a garnish.

61. Delicious Muffin Snack

INGREDIENTS | **Servings:** 2
- ½ cup tomato sauce
- 4 muffins
- 1 red capsicum, sliced
- oregano leaves to garnish
- 2 cups ricotta
- 1 tbsp. capers

DIRECTIONS | **Ready in about:** 20 min

Add tomato sauce into the air fryer pot. Combine the red capsicum, capers and ricotta. Cook at 300°F for 15 minutes. When finished, apply the mixture to the muffins. Garnish with oregano leaves for serving!

62. Grilled Cheese Delight

INGREDIENTS | **Servings:** 2
- ¼ cup butter, melted
- 4 slices white bread
- ½ cup sharp cheddar cheese

DIRECTIONS | **Ready in about:** 15 min

Warm the air fryer to 360°F. Place butter and cheese in two separate containers. Brush the butter on both sides of the bread. Put the cheese on 2 of the 4 pieces of bread. Add the grilled cheese and add it to the cooking basket of the air fryer. Bake until cheese is melted and golden, or 5 to 7 minutes.

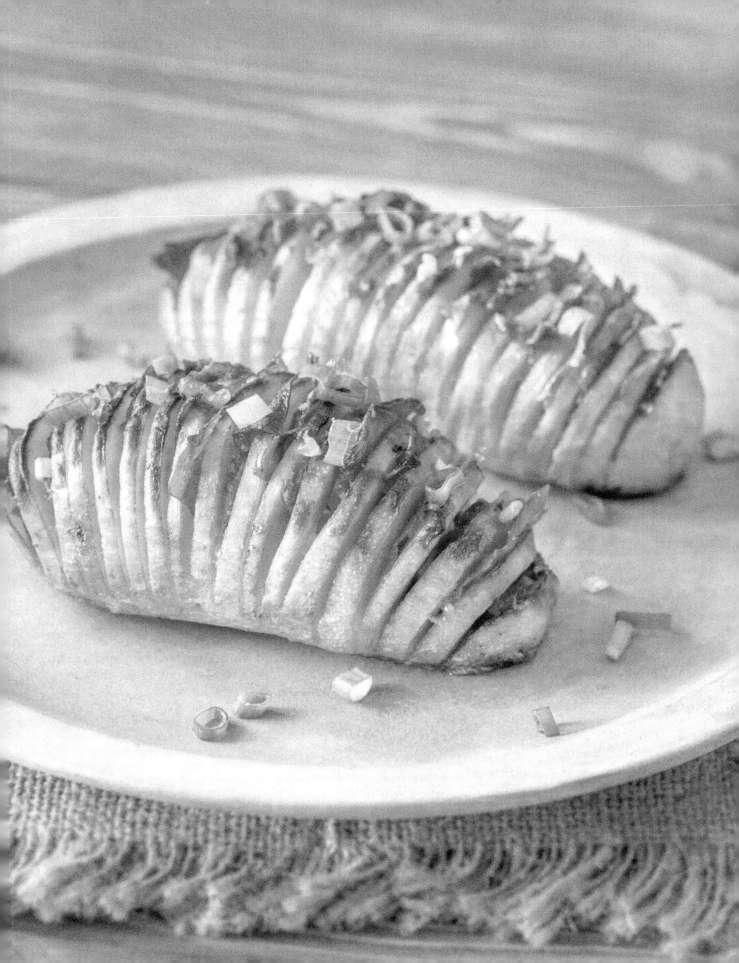

63. Hasselback Potatoes

INGREDIENTS | **Servings:** 2
- 2 tbsp. olive oil
- 2 potatoes, peeled and thinly sliced almost all the way horizontally
- 1 tsp. garlic, minced
- ½ tsp. oregano, dried
- ½ tsp. sweet paprika
- salt and black pepper to taste
- ½ tsp. basil, dried

DIRECTIONS | **Ready in about:** 30 min

In a bowl, combine the oil with the garlic, salt, pepper, oregano, basil and paprika and mix well. Rub the potatoes with this mixture, put them in the basket of your air fryer and fry them at 350°F for 20 minutes. Divide them among plates and serve as a garnish.

64. Nutella Mix Snack

INGREDIENTS | **Servings:** 2
- 2 tbsp. Nutella
- 4 pizza snack plates
- 1 small packet pikelets
- 2 tbsp. vanilla frosting

DIRECTIONS | **Ready in about:** 20 min

Add the pikelets to the air fryer. Mix the icing on Nutella and vanilla. Bake at 300°F for 5 minutes. When finished, apply the mixture to the pizza plates to serve!

65. Nuts Mix Snack

INGREDIENTS | **Servings:** 2
- 2 tbsp. oil
- 1 tbsp. garlic clove (minced)
- 1 tbsp. paprika
- 3 tbsp. chili powder
- salt to taste
- 3 cup macadamia nuts
- 3 cup cashew nuts
- 1 tbsp. almond kernels
- 1 cup brazil nuts

DIRECTIONS | **Ready in about:** 15 min

Mix oil into the air fryer pot. Add the garlic clove, chili powder, paprika, salt, a hazelnut almond, cashews, Brazil nuts and macadamia nuts. Bake at 300°F for 10 minutes. When you are ready, help yourself and enjoy!

66. Puff Pastry Appetizer

INGREDIENTS | **Servings:** 2
- 1 tbsp. oil
- 1 onion, chopped
- salt to taste
- 3 tbsp. cumin seeds
- 1 tbsp. turmeric powder
- 3 tsp. chili powder
- 1 garlic clove, minced
- 2 potatoes, mashed
- 1 tbsp. lemon juice
- 3 cup parsley, chopped
- 3 sheets puff pastry
- 2 eggs

DIRECTIONS | **Ready in about:** 20 min

Add oil and onion into the air fryer pot. Combine the salt, cumin seeds, turmeric powder, chili powder, garlic, potatoes, lemon juice, eggs and parsley. Bake at 300°F for 15 minutes. Put the puff pastry on top of the mixture and cook for another 5 minutes. When it's ready, serve!

67. Spring Onion Mix Snack

INGREDIENTS | **Servings:** 2
- 1 cup cheddar cheese
- 3 cup sour cream
- 3 cup flour
- 1 red capsicum, diced
- 2 spring onions, sliced
- 2 eggs
- 2 tbsp. butter
- chives to garnish

DIRECTIONS | **Ready in about:** 20 min

Add the eggs and flour to a portable bowl. Add sour cream, red pepper, chives and butter. Pour the mixture into the round baking pan. Bake at 300°F for 15 minutes. When cooked, garnish with chives and cheddar cheese for serving.

68. Sundried Tomatoes Snack

INGREDIENTS | **Servings:** 2

- 2 tbsp. butter
- 2 cups sundried tomatoes
- 2 tbsp. paprika
- 1 tbsp. oregano
- salt to taste

DIRECTIONS | **Ready in about:** 14 min

Add butter into the air fryer pot. Combine the sundried tomatoes, paprika, oregano and salt. Bake at 300°F for 10 minutes. When it's ready, serve!

69. Sweet Potato Fries

INGREDIENTS | **Servings:** 2

- salt and black pepper to taste
- 2 sweet potatoes, peeled and cut into medium fries
- 2 tbsp. olive oil
- ¼ tsp. coriander, ground
- ½ tsp. curry powder
- ¼ cup ketchup
- 1 pinch of cinnamon powder
- ½ tsp. cumin, ground
- 2 tbsp. mayonnaise
- 1 pinch of ginger powder

DIRECTIONS | **Ready in about:** 30 min

In the air fryer basket, mixing the chips with salt, pepper, coriander, curry powder, and the oil well mix and cook at 370°F for 20 minutes, turning once. Meanwhile, in a bowl, combine the ketchup with mayonnaise, cumin, ginger, and cinnamon and mix well. Divide the fries between plates, pour the tomato sauce mixture over them, and serve as a garnish. Enjoy!

70. Tortillas with Banana

INGREDIENTS | **Servings:** 2

- 2 tbsp. fresh ricotta
- 1 tbsp. honey
- 2 mini tortillas
- 1 banana, sliced

DIRECTIONS | **Ready in about:** 10 min

Add honey into the air fryer pot. Stir in the fresh ricotta and banana. Add the tortillas. Bake at 250°F for 5 minutes. When you're ready, help yourself and enjoy the crunchy appetizer!

71. Yellow Squash and Zucchinis

INGREDIENTS | **Servings:** 2

- 1 tbsp. tarragon, chopped
- salt and white pepper to taste
- 1 yellow squash, halved, deseeded and cut into chunks
- 1-pound zucchinis, sliced
- 6 tsp. olive oil
- ½ pound carrots, cubed

DIRECTIONS | **Ready in about:** 45 min

In your air fryer basket, toss zucchini with carrots, squash, salt, pepper and oil, mix well and cook at 400°F for 25 minutes. Divide them among plates and serve as a garnish with a pinch of tarragon.

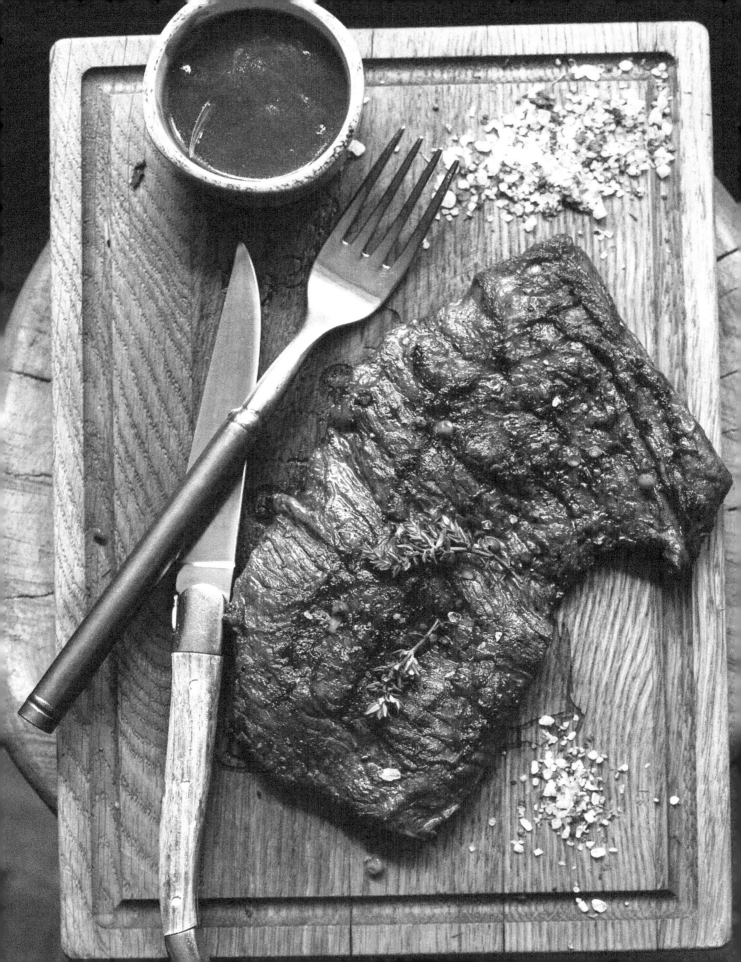

BEEF, PORK, & LAMB

72. Amazing Beef Balls

INGREDIENTS | **Servings:** 2
- 1 lb. beef balls (frozen)
- 1 tbsp. dill
- 1 tbsp. onion powder
- 1 cup parsley
- 2 tbsp. paprika
- 1 tbsp. garlic powder
- 1 tbsp. lemon pepper
- 2 tbsp. lemon juice

DIRECTIONS | **Ready in about:** 15 min

Add onion powder and parsley into the air fryer. Combine the dill, paprika, garlic powder, pepper and lemon juice. Place the beef meatballs in the pot. Cook at 300°F for 10 minutes. When it's ready, help yourself and enjoy!

73. Bacon Mixed

INGREDIENTS | **Servings:** 2
- 3 tbsp. lemon juice
- 2 tbsp. olive oil
- ½ cup cilantro, chopped
- salt and pepper to taste
- ½ cup cilantro
- 1 lb. shrimp, pieces
- 4 bacon slices
- 2 avocados, cubed
- 4 cups lettuce, chopped

DIRECTIONS | **Ready in about:** 25 min

Add oil into the air fryer pot. Combine the lemon juice, cilantro, shrimp, bacon slices with salt and pepper. Cook at 300°F for 20 minutes. Meanwhile, whisk together the avocado, lettuce and cilantro sauce. When it's ready, help yourself and enjoy!

74. Bacon with Mustard

INGREDIENTS | **Servings:** 2
- 1 tbsp. Dijon mustard
- 2 strips Bacon
- ½ lb. Pork tenderloin

DIRECTIONS | **Ready in about:** 45 min

Set the air-fryer temperature to 360°F. Sprinkle mustard over steak and wrap in bacon. Air fry them for 15 minutes. Overturn and cook for an additional 10 to 15 minutes. Serve with your favorite sides.

75. Bacon-Wrapped Hot Dog

INGREDIENTS | **Servings:** 2
- 2 beef hot dogs
- 2 slices sugar-free bacon

DIRECTIONS | **Ready in about:** 15 min

Swathe each hot dog with a slice of bacon and secure it with a toothpick. Place in the air fryer basket. Set the temperature to 370°F and set the timer for 10 minutes. Turn each hot dog halfway through cooking. When cooked, the bacon will be crisp. Serve hot.

76. Beef and Pork Mix

INGREDIENTS | **Servings:** 2
- 1 onion, chopped
- ⅔ pound beef, grounded
- ⅓ pound pork, grounded
- salt and pepper to taste
- ¼ tsp. nutmeg
- ¼ tsp. ginger powder
- 2 cups beef broth
- ½ cup sour cream

DIRECTIONS | **Ready in about:** 35 min

Add beef broth into the air fryer pot. Combine the ginger, nutmeg, salt, pepper and onion. Add the beef and pork. Bake at 400°F for 30 minutes. Serve with sour cream when it's done.

77. Beef Breast Pieces with Celery

INGREDIENTS | **Servings:** 2

- 2 tbsp. butter
- 1 cup onion, chopped
- 1 cup celery, chopped
- 1 beef broth, can
- 2 lb. beef breast piece, chunks
- 1 vegetable broth, can
- 2 cup sliced carrots
- 1 tsp. basil
- 1 tsp. oregano
- salt and pepper to taste

DIRECTIONS | **Ready in about:** 35 min

Season the artichokes with salt and pepper, rub them with half the oil and half the lemon juice, put them in your air fryer and cook at 360°F for 7 minutes. Meanwhile, in a bowl, combine the remaining lemon juice with the vinegar, remaining oil, salt, pepper, garlic and oregano and mix well. Arrange the artichokes on a serving platter, sprinkle with balsamic vinaigrette and serve.

78. Beef Loaf with Black Olives

INGREDIENTS | **Servings:** 2

- 1 lb. beef loaf
- 2 tbsp. oil
- 2 tomatoes, chopped
- ½ cup Peas
- 1 cup basil, chopped
- 2 cups cheese, shredded
- 1 onion, chopped
- ½ cup black olives
- 2 tbsp. lemon Juice
- salt and pepper to taste

DIRECTIONS | **Ready in about:** 30 min

Add oil into the air fryer pot. Mix the tomatoes, peas, basil, cheese, onions, black olives, lemon juice with salt and pepper. Add the beef loaf. Cook at 300°F for 25 minutes. When you're ready, serve!

79. Beef Mix Carrot

INGREDIENTS | **Servings:** 2

- 2 pounds beef, grounded
- ½ cup onion, chopped
- ½ tsp. ginger powder
- salt and pepper to taste
- 2 tsp. sugar
- 3 tbsp. vinegar
- 1 tbsp. soy sauce
- ½ tsp. ginger powder
- 1 large carrot
- 1 large green bell pepper

DIRECTIONS | **Ready in about:** 30 min

Add beef into the air fryer pot. Combine soy sauce, vinegar, ground ginger, salt and pepper, and ground ginger. Cook at 300°F for 15 minutes. Add the green pepper and carrots. Cook for another 10 minutes.

80. Beef Steak Delight

INGREDIENTS | **Servings:** 2

- 1 lb. beef steaks
- 4 tbsp. lemon juice
- 2 tbsp. butter
- 2 garlic cloves
- ½ cup parsley
- salt and pepper to taste

DIRECTIONS | **Ready in about:** 26 min

Add butter into the air fryer pot. Mix the lemon juice, garlic, parsley with salt and pepper. Add the beef steaks. Cook at 300°F for 20 minutes. 5. Serve and enjoy!

81. Beef Steak with Tomato Soup

INGREDIENTS | **Servings:** 2

- 4 beef steaks
- 1 tsp. butter
- 14 ounces broth of beef
- 10 ounces tomato soup
- 1½ cup water
- 3 cups cabbage, shredded
- 1 onion, chopped
- ½ cup green bell pepper, diced
- salt and pepper to taste

DIRECTIONS | **Ready in about:** 24 min

Add beef steaks into the air fryer pot. Combine butter, broth, tomato soup, water, cabbage, onion, green pepper with salt and pepper. Cook at 300°F for 20 minutes. When it's ready, help yourself and enjoy!

82. Beef Strips with Snow Peas and Mushrooms

INGREDIENTS | **Servings:** 2

- salt and black pepper to taste
- 2 beef steaks, cut into strips
- 7 ounces snow peas
- 1 yellow onion, cut into rings
- 1 tsp. olive oil
- 8 ounces white mushrooms, halved
- 2 tbsp. soy sauce

DIRECTIONS | **Ready in about:** 25 min

In a portable bowl, mix the olive oil with the soy sauce, beat, add the beef strips and mix. In another bowl, mix the peas, onion and mushrooms with salt, pepper and oil, mix well, put in a saucepan suitable for your air fryer and bake at 350°F for 16 minutes. The beef strips also be added the meat in the pan and bake at 400°F for 6 minutes more. Divide everything between plates and serve.

83. Beef Stuffed Squash

INGREDIENTS | **Servings:** 2

- 1 pound beef, ground
- 1 spaghetti squash, pricked
- salt and black pepper to the taste
- 1 yellow onion, chopped
- 3 garlic cloves, minced
- 1 Portobello mushroom, sliced
- 1 tsp. oregano, dried
- 28 ounces canned tomatoes, chopped
- ¼ tsp. cayenne pepper
- 1 green bell pepper, chopped
- ½ tsp. thyme, dried

DIRECTIONS | **Ready in about:** 50 min

Place the spaghetti in the air fryer, cook at 350°F for 20 minutes, transfer to a cutting board, cut in half and discard the seeds. Heat a pan over medium-high heat, add the meat, garlic, onion and mushrooms, stir and cook until the meat is golden brown. Add salt, pepper, thyme, oregano, cayenne pepper, tomatoes and the green peppers, mix and cook 10 minutes. Stuff squash with this beef mix, place it in the fryer and cook at 360°F for 10 minutes. Divide into plates and serve.

84. Beef with Arugula

INGREDIENTS | **Servings:** 2

- 1 lb. beef, chopped
- 1 bunch parsley, chopped
- 1 tsp. Dijon mustard
- salt and pepper to taste
- 2 cups arugula
- 1 lemon juice
- 1 tsp. white vinegar
- 1 tbsp. olive oil

DIRECTIONS | **Ready in about:** 35 min

Add oil into the air fryer pot. Combine beef, parsley, Dijon mustard, arugula, lemon juice, white vinegar with salt and pepper. Cook at 300°F for 30 minutes. Serve and enjoy!

85. Beef with Cheese Mix

INGREDIENTS | **Servings:** 2

- 3 garlic cloves
- 1 cup cheddar cheese
- 2 lb. grounded beef
- 2 tsp. dried oregano
- 2 tbsp. olive oil
- 1 pinch dried chili flakes
- 2 chopped tomatoes

DIRECTIONS | **Ready in about:** 26 min

Add beef into the air fryer pot. Toss the garlic cloves, dried oregano, chili flakes and diced tomatoes with the minced meat. Cook at 300°F for 20 minutes. When you're ready, top the cheese for serving!

86. Beef with Corn Kernels

INGREDIENTS | **Servings:** 2
- 2 cups corn kernels
- 2 onions, chopped)
- ½ cup Jicama
- ½ cup bell pepper
- 1 cup cilantro leaves
- ½ cup lemon juice
- salt and pepper to taste
- 1 lb. beef
- 1 tbsp. oil
- 5 corn tortillas
- 2 tbsp. sour cream

DIRECTIONS | **Ready in about:** 25 min

Add Jicama and oil into the air fryer pot. Mix the corn, onions, peppers, cilantro, lemon juice, sour cream and beef with salt and pepper. Cook at 300°F for 20 minutes. When it's ready, top the tortillas with corn for serving!

87. Beef with Linguine

INGREDIENTS | **Servings:** 2
- 1 pound linguine
- 1 tbsp. butter
- ½ cup white wine
- 1 lb. grounded beef
- 1 cup cheese, shredded
- 2 garlic cloves, minced
- 1 cup parsley
- salt and pepper to taste
- 1 lb. shrimps, cleaned

DIRECTIONS | **Ready in about:** 25 min

Add butter into the air fryer pot. Mix linguine, white wine, minced meat, cheese, garlic, parsley, shrimp with salt and pepper. Cook at 300°F for 20 minutes. Serve and enjoy!

88. Beef with Mushrooms

INGREDIENTS | **Servings:** 2
- ¼ cup oil
- 1 bell pepper
- 1 onion, chopped
- 2 cups beef, chopped, breast
- 4½ ounce Mushrooms
- 4½ ounce tomatoes, diced
- 3 garlic cloves
- 1 tsp. soy sauce
- salt and pepper to taste
- 3 drops hot sauce

DIRECTIONS | **Ready in about:** 25 min

Add oil into the air fryer pot. Mix the bell pepper, onion, meat, mushrooms, tomatoes, garlic, soy sauce, hot sauce with salt and pepper. Bake at 300°F for 20 minutes. When it's, help yourself and enjoy!

89. Beef with Mushrooms and Onions

INGREDIENTS | **Servings:** 2
- 1 lb. beef
- 2 potatoes, cubed
- 2 onions, chopped
- 1 tbsp. butter
- 1 cup mushrooms
- salt and pepper to taste
- 1 tbsp. lemon juice

DIRECTIONS | **Ready in about:** 25 min

Add butter into the air fryer pot. Combine the beef, potatoes, onions, mushrooms, lemon juice with salt and pepper. Cook at 300°F for 20 minutes. When it's ready, help yourself and enjoy!

90. Beef with Potatoes

INGREDIENTS | **Servings:** 2
- 4 large beef steak pieces
- 10 potatoes, cubed
- 8 ounces carrots
- 1 cup celery, chopped
- 2 beef soup cans
- 2 tsp. garlic salt
- 1 tsp. celery salt
- black pepper to taste
- 1 small bag mixed vegetables (frozen)

DIRECTIONS | **Ready in about:** 25 min

Add potatoes into the air fryer pot. Combine carrots, celery, canned beef soup, salt, garlic salt, celery, black pepper and a mixture of vegetables. Add the beef steaks. Cook at 300°F for 20 minutes. Serve and enjoy!

91. Beef Worcestershire

INGREDIENTS | **Servings:** 2

- ½ cup balsamic vinegar
- ¼ cup soy sauce
- 3 tbsp. garlic, chopped
- 2 tbsp. honey
- salt and pepper to taste
- 1 tsp. Worcestershire sauce
- 1 tsp. onion powder
- 1 tsp. smoke flavor liquid
- 1 pinch Cayenne pepper
- 2 ½ pound beef steaks

DIRECTIONS | **Ready in about:** 25 min

Add garlic and soy sauce into the air fryer pot. Mix the balsamic vinegar, soy sauce, honey, salt and pepper, Worcestershire sauce, onion powder and pepper Cayenne powder. Mix well. Add the beefsteak. Pour the mixture over it. Cook at 350°F for 20 minutes. When it's done, remove it and serve it!

92. Buttered Striploin Steak

INGREDIENTS | **Servings:** 2

- 2 (7 ounces) striploin steak
- 1½ tbsp. butter, softened
- salt and black pepper, to taste

DIRECTIONS | **Ready in about:** 22 min

Warm up the air fryer to 390°F and grease the air fryer basket. Liberally rub the steak with salt and black pepper and cover with butter. Transfer the steak to the air fryer basket and cook for about 12 minutes, turning it once in the middle. Serve the steak and slice it to the desired size for serving.

93. Air Fried Cheeseburgers

INGREDIENTS | **Servings:** 2

- 2 bread rolls
- 2 slices of cheddar cheese
- ½ pound of ground beef
- 2 tsp. of salt
- 2 tbsp. of melted butter
- ½ tsp. of black pepper, ground

DIRECTIONS | **Ready in about:** 15 min

Heat the air fryer to 390°F. Shaping ground beef to form 2 meatballs. Sprinkle with salt and pepper. Cut the sandwiches in the center and place each burger in them. Place the burgers in the cooking basket and cook for about 11 minutes. Add the cheddar cheese to the meatballs and cook 1 minute longer until the cheese is melted.

94. Comforting Sausage Casserole

INGREDIENTS | **Servings:** 2

- 2 eggs
- 6 ounces flour
- 1 red onion, sliced thinly
- 8 small sausages
- ¾ cup milk
- 1 tbsp. olive oil
- salt and black pepper, to taste
- 1 garlic clove, mince

DIRECTIONS | **Ready in about:** 45 min

Warm up the air fryer to 320°F and grease a saucepan. Sift the flour into a bowl and beat the eggs. Mix well and add the onion, garlic, milk, ⅔ cup cold water, salt and the pepper black. Pierce 1 sprig of rosemary in each sausage and transfer to the pot. Sprinkle evenly with the flour mixture and cook for about 30 minutes. Dish out and serve hot.

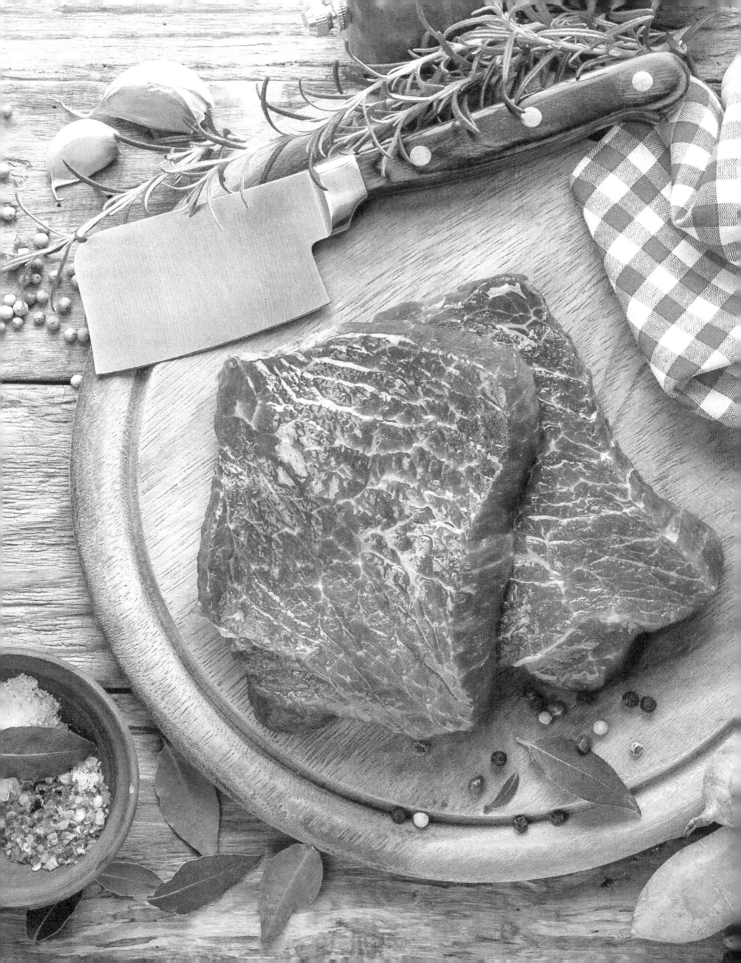

95. Crispy Pork Chop Salad

INGREDIENTS | **Servings:** 2

- 2 (4 ounces) pork chops, chopped into 1" cubes
- 1 tbsp. coconut oil
- 2 tsp. chili powder
- ½ tsp. garlic powder
- 1 tsp. paprika
- ¼ tsp. onion powder
- 1 tbsp. chopped cilantro
- Monterey jack cheese
- 4 cups chopped romaine
- ½ cup shredded
- 1 medium Roma tomato, diced
- 1 medium avocado, peeled, pitted, and diced
- ¼ cup full-fat ranch dressing

DIRECTIONS | **Ready in about:** 23 min

In an enormous bowl, pour the coconut oil over the pork. Sprinkle with chili powder, paprika, garlic powder and onion powder. Place the pork in the air fryer basket. Set the temperature to 400°F and set the timer for 8 minutes. The pork will be brown and crispy when fully cooked. In an enormous bowl, place the romaine lettuce, tomato and crispy pork. Garnish with grated cheese and avocado. Pour the ranch dressing around the bowl and toss the salad to coat well. Garnish with cilantro. Serve immediately.

96. Easy Juicy Pork Chops

INGREDIENTS | **Servings:** 2

- ½ tsp. garlic powder
- 1 tsp. chili powder
- 1/2 tsp. cumin
- 2 tbsp. unsalted butter, divided
- ¼ tsp. dried oregano
- ¼ tsp. ground black pepper
- 2 (4 ounces) boneless pork chops

DIRECTIONS | **Ready in about:** 20 min

In a portable bowl, combine the chili powder, garlic powder, cumin, pepper and oregano. Dry rub the pork ribs. Place the pork chops in the basket of the air fryer. Set the temperature to 400°F and set the timer for 15 minutes. Core temperature should be at least 145°F when fully cooked. Serve hot, garnished with a tbsp. of butter.

97. Ground Beef with Spinach Leaves

INGREDIENTS | **Servings:** 2

- 1 lb. ground beef
- 1 onion, chopped
- 2 cloves garlic, minced
- 2 cups tomato sauce
- 1 tbsp. Worcestershire sauce
- cheese to dress
- 2 cups beef broth
- 2 diced tomatoes
- 3 bunch chopped spinach leaves
- salt and pepper to taste

DIRECTIONS | **Ready in about:** 42 min

Add beef broth into the air fryer pot. Combine onion, garlic, ketchup, Worcestershire sauce and tomato. Add the meat and cook for 15 minutes. My spinach leaves with salt and pepper. Cook at 300°F for another 20 minutes. Serve with a pinch of cheese when it's ready.

98. Grounded Beef with Bacon

INGREDIENTS | **Servings:** 2

- 1 pound spaghetti, boiled
- 1 tbsp. olive oil
- 8 diced bacon slices
- 1 onion, chopped
- 1 garlic clove, minced
- ½ cup Parmesan cheese, grated
- salt and pepper to taste
- 2 tbsp. fresh parsley, chopped
- 2 lb. grounded beef

DIRECTIONS | **Ready in about:** 15 min

Add oil into the air fryer pot. Toss bacon slices, onion, garlic, Parmesan, parsley beef with salt and pepper. Cook at 300°F for 10 minutes. Add the spaghetti and cook for another 10 minutes. When it's ready, help yourself and enjoy!

99. Grounded Beef with Pork and Veal

INGREDIENTS | **Servings:** 2

- 1-pound grounded beef
- ½ pound veal, grounded
- ½ pound pork, grounded
- salt and pepper to taste
- ⅓ cup onion, chopped
- 2 cups sour cream
- ¼ cup fresh dill

DIRECTIONS | **Ready in about:** 20 min

Add onion into the air fryer pot. Combine fresh dill, flour, butter, cream, onion, pork, beef and ground beef. Cook at 300°F for 15 minutes. When it's ready, serve it with sour cream and enjoy your meal!

100. Grounded Beef with Rice

INGREDIENTS | **Servings:** 2

- 3 cups shrimps
- 2 chopped tomatoes
- 2 cups chopped olives
- 2 tbsp. capers
- 1 cup chopped thyme
- salt and pepper to taste
- 2 cups white rice, boiled
- 1 lb. grounded beef

DIRECTIONS | **Ready in about:** 25 min

Add tomatoes and shrimps into the air fryer pot. Mix the olives, capers, thyme, white rice with salt and pepper. Add the ground beef. Cook at 300°F for 20 minutes. When it's ready, serve!

101. Grounded Pork with Carrots and Rice

INGREDIENTS | **Servings:** 2

- 1 lb. ground pork sausage
- 5 beaten eggs
- 3 tbsp. vegetable oil
- ½ cored and shredded cabbage
- 3 finely chopped carrots
- 6 cups cold, cooked white rice
- ¼ cup soy sauce
- 1 frozen package of 6 ounces thawed, green pea
- 1 package of 14½ ounces drained, can bean sprouts
- 3 finely chopped onions
- salt and pepper to taste

DIRECTIONS | **Ready in about:** 25 min

Add vegetable oil into the air fryer pot. Mix the pork sausage with cabbage, carrot, white rice, soy sauce, peas, bean sprouts, onion with salt and pepper. Cook at 300°F for 20 minutes. When it's ready, help yourself and enjoy!

102. Maple Syrup Mix Beef

INGREDIENTS | **Servings:** 2

- ½ cup soy sauce
- ¼ cup maple syrup
- 6 cloves garlic, chopped
- 1 tbsp. ginger, grated
- 1 tsp. mustard powder
- 1 tsp. sesame oil
- ¼ tsp. hot pepper sauce
- ½ cup beer
- 4 (10 ounces) beef steak

DIRECTIONS | **Ready in about:** 20 min

Add sesame oil into the air fryer pot. Combine soy sauce, garlic, ginger, mustard powder, hot sauce, maple syrup and beer in the bowl. Add the beef steak to the pot. Pour the mixture over it. Cook at 400°F for 15 minutes. Serve when it's ready!

103. Mediterranean Steaks and Scallops

INGREDIENTS | **Servings:** 2

- 2 beef steaks
- 10 sea scallops
- 4 garlic cloves, minced
- 2 tbsp. lemon juice
- 1 shallot, chopped
- 2 tbsp. parsley, chopped
- 1 tsp. lemon zest
- 2 tbsp. basil, chopped
- ¼ cup butter
- salt and black pepper to the taste
- ¼ cup veggie stock

DIRECTIONS | **Ready in about:** 25 min

Spice the steaks with salt and pepper, place them in the air fryer, cook at 360°F for 10 minutes and transfer them to an air fryer. Add shallot, garlic, butter, broth, basil, lemon juice, parsley, the zest of lemon and scallops, stir gently and cook at 360°F for another 4 minutes. Divide the steaks and scallops between plates and serve.

104. Pork Chops and Sage Sauce

INGREDIENTS | **Servings:** 2
- salt and black pepper to taste
- 2 pork chops
- 1 tbsp. olive oil
- 1 tsp. lemon juice
- 1 shallot, sliced
- 2 tbsp. butter
- 1 handful sage, chopped

DIRECTIONS | **Ready in about:** 25 min

Spice the pork chops with salt and pepper, rub in oil, put in the air fryer and cook at 370°F for 10 minutes, turning them halfway. Meanwhile, make heat a frying pan with the butter over medium heat, add shallots, stir and cook for 2 minutes. Add sage and lemon juice, mix well, cook for a few more minutes and remove from heat. Divide the pork chops between plates, sprinkle with sage sauce and serve.

105. Pork with Black Olives

INGREDIENTS | **Servings:** 2
- 1lb. pork
- 2 tbsp. oil
- 2 tomatoes
- ½ cup peas
- 1 cup basil, chopped
- 2 cups cheese, shredded
- 1 onion, chopped
- ½ cup black olives, small pieces
- 2 tbsp. lemon juice
- salt and pepper to taste

DIRECTIONS | **Ready in about:** 19 min

Add oil into the air fryer pot. Mix the pork with the lemon juice. Add the tomatoes, peas, basil, onion, black olives with salt and pepper. Cook at 300°F for 15 minutes. Serve and enjoy!

106. Pork with Honey Mix

INGREDIENTS | **Servings:** 2
- ½ tsp. red pepper
- ½ tsp. ginger powder
- ¼ tsp. vegetable oil
- 2 onions
- 2 garlic cloves
- 2 tbsp. ketchup
- 1 tbsp. soy sauce
- 2 tbsp. cornstarch
- 1 tsp. honey
- 1 lb. pork, cubed

DIRECTIONS | **Ready in about:** 36 min

Add ketchup and soy sauce into the air fryer pot. Mix cornstarch, honey, chilli, ginger powder, oil, onions, garlic and pork. Cook at 300°F for 30 minutes. When it's ready, help yourself and enjoy!

107. Pork with White Rice

INGREDIENTS | **Servings:** 2
- 1 lb. pork, chopped
- 2 cups white rice
- 1 tbsp. cayenne powder
- 2 tbsp. chili powder
- salt and pepper to taste
- 2 cups beef broth
- 2 garlic cloves, minced

DIRECTIONS | **Ready in about:** 26 min

Add pork and beef broth into the air fryer pot. Combine white rice, cayenne pepper powder, chili powder, garlic from the salt and pepper. Cook at 300°F for 20 minutes. Serve and enjoy it when it's ready.

108. Provencal Pork

INGREDIENTS | **Servings:** 2
- 1 yellow bell pepper, cut into strips
- 1 red onion, sliced
- 1 green bell pepper, cut into strips
- 2 tsp. Provencal herbs
- salt and black pepper to taste
- ½ tbsp. mustard
- 7 ounces pork tenderloin
- 1 tbsp. olive oil

DIRECTIONS | **Ready in about:** 25 min

In a baking dish suitable for your air fryer, mix the yellow pepper with the green pepper, onion, salt, pepper, Provence herbs and half the oil and mix well. Season the pork with salt, pepper, mustard and the rest of the oil, mix well and add to the vegetables. Put everything in your air fryer, bake at 370°F for 15 minutes, divide between plates and serve.

109. Quick Beef

INGREDIENTS | Servings: 2
- 1 tbsp. canola oil
- ¼ cup ground beef
- 1 sliced green onion, separated green and white parts
- 3 cups short grain rice, cooked
- 1 tsp. sesame oil
- 1 tsp. butter
- 1 egg

DIRECTIONS | Ready in about: 25 min

Add canola oil into the air fryer pot. Combine the green onion, sesame oil, butter and egg. Add the ground beef and rice. Bake at 300°F for 20 minutes. When it's ready, serve!

110. Red Meat Delight

INGREDIENTS | Servings: 2
- 1 lb. red meat
- 4 tbsp. lemon juice
- 2 tbsp. butter
- 2 garlic cloves
- ½ cup parsley
- salt and pepper to taste

DIRECTIONS | Ready in about: 25 min

Add butter into the air fryer pot. Mix the lemon juice, red half, garlic cloves, parsley with salt and pepper. Cook at 400°F for 20 minutes. When it's ready, help yourself and enjoy!

111. Reverse Seared Ribeye

INGREDIENTS | Servings: 2
- ½ tsp. pink Himalayan salt
- 1 (8 ounces) ribeye steak
- ¼ tsp. ground peppercorn
- 1 tbsp. salted butter, softened
- 1 tbsp. coconut oil
- ¼ tsp. garlic powder
- ¼ tsp. dried oregano
- ½ tsp. dried parsley

DIRECTIONS | Ready in about: 50 min

Rub the steak with salt and ground pepper. Place it in the air fryer basket. Set the temperature to 250°F and set the timer for 45 minutes. Once the timer is off, start checking doneness and add a few minutes until core temperature is your personal preference. In a standard skillet over medium heat, add the coconut or the. When the oil is hot, quickly sear the outside and sides of the steak until it is crisp and golden. Remove from the heat and let the fillet rest. In a small bowl, beat the butter with the garlic powder, parsley and oregano. Slices the steak and serve with the herb butter on top.

112. Scallops with Beef Special

INGREDIENTS | Servings: 2
- 1 lb. scallops
- 1 lb. beef
- 2 onions, chopped
- 1 tbsp. butter
- 1 cup mushrooms
- 1 tbsp. lemon juice
- salt and pepper to taste

DIRECTIONS | Ready in about: 24 min

Add beef and scallops into the air fryer pot. Mix the onions, butter, mushrooms, lemon juice with salt and pepper. Cook at 300°F for 20 minutes. Serve and enjoy!

113. Shrimp and Beef with Lettuce

INGREDIENTS | Servings: 2
- 3 tbsp. lemon juice
- 2 tbsp. olive oil
- ½ cup cilantro, chopped
- 1 lb. beef
- salt and pepper to taste
- ½ cup cilantro dressing
- 1 lb. shrimp, pieces
- 2 avocados
- 4 cups lettuce

DIRECTIONS | Ready in about: 19 min

Add olive oil into the air fryer pot. Toss the shrimp with salt, pepper and lemon juice. Add the meat. Bake at 300°F for 20 minutes. Meanwhile, combine avocado, lettuce and cilantro in a bowl. When you are ready, serve the meat with the avocado and cilantro mixture.

114. Shrimps and Red Meat Mix

INGREDIENTS | **Servings:** 2
- 1 lb. shrimps
- 2 garlic cloves
- 2 tbsp. oil
- 1 lb. red meat, sliced
- 2 cups white rice, boiled
- salt and pepper to taste
- 1 cup parsley, chopped

DIRECTIONS | **Ready in about:** 19 min

Add oil into the air fryer pot. Mix the red meat, garlic, shrimp, parsley with salt and pepper. Cook at 300°F for 20 minutes. Add the rice. Cook for another 10 minutes. When it's ready, help yourself and enjoy!

115. Shrimps with Honey and Beef

INGREDIENTS | **Servings:** 2
- 2 tbsp. ketchup
- 1 tbsp. soy sauce
- 2 tbsp. cornstarch
- 1 tsp. honey
- ½ tsp. red pepper
- ½ tsp. ginger powder
- ¼ tsp. vegetable oil
- 2 onions
- 2 garlic cloves
- 1 lb. shrimps, tails removed
- 1 lb. beef, cubed

DIRECTIONS | **Ready in about:** 25 min

Add honey and ketchup into the air fryer pot. Combine soy sauce, cornstarch, red pepper, ginger powder, oil, garlic, onion and shrimp. Add the beef. Cook at 300°F for 20 minutes. When it's ready, help yourself and enjoy!

116. Simply Beef and Shrimp

INGREDIENTS | **Servings:** 2
- 1 lb. shrimps
- 1 lb. beef, sliced
- 2 garlic cloves
- 2 tbsp. oil
- 1 tbsp. butter
- red pepper as needed
- salt and pepper to taste
- 1 cup parsley, chopped

DIRECTIONS | **Ready in about:** 25 min

Add oil into the air fryer pot. Combine the garlic cloves, meat, shrimp, butter, chili, parsley with salt and pepper. Cook at 300°F for 20 minutes. Serve and enjoy!

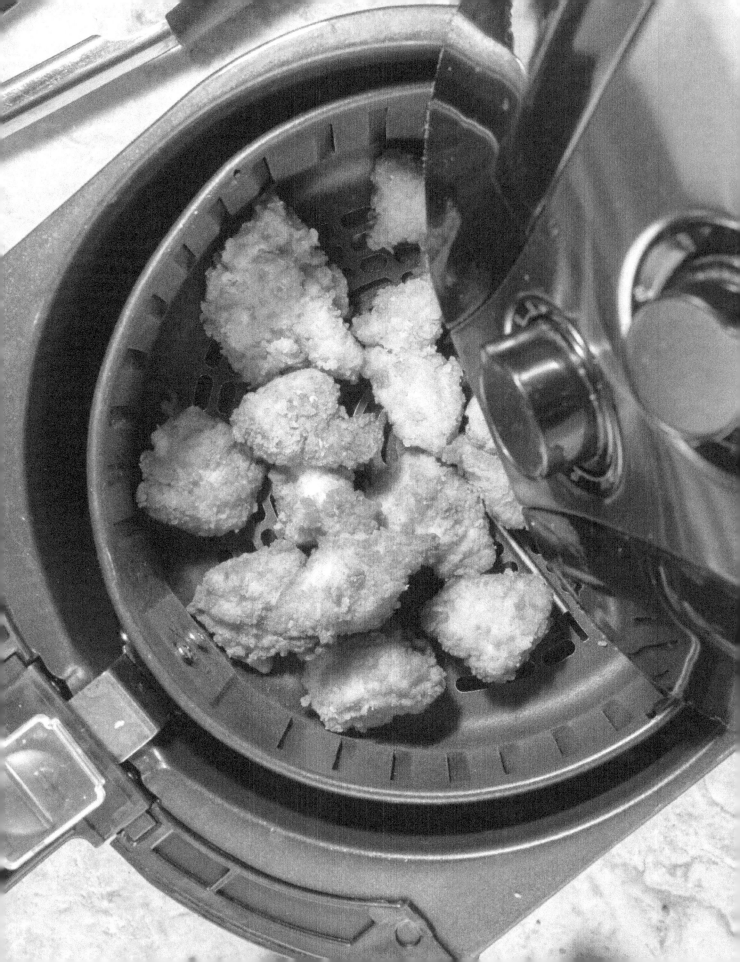

POULTRY

117. Buffalo Chicken Meatballs

INGREDIENTS | **Servings:** 2
- 4 garlic cloves
- 1-pound ground chicken
- 1 package ranch seasoning
- 1 cup ranch dressing
- 1 cup seasoned breadcrumbs
- 1 cup hot sauce
- ½ cup blue cheese crumbles

DIRECTIONS | **Ready in about:** 20 min

Chop the garlic. Combine garlic, ranch dressing and breadcrumbs in a large bowl. Add the chicken and bring the ingredients together on their knees. Roll into balls. Bake at 360°F for 5 minutes. Stir the meatballs into the hot sauce and cook for another 5 minutes. Combine ranch cheese and crumbled blue cheese. Sprinkle ranch mixture over meatballs before serving.

118. Buffalo Wings

INGREDIENTS | **Servings:** 2
- 1 tbsp. butter, melted
- 14 ounces chicken wings
- 2 tsp. cayenne pepper
- 2 tbsp. red hot sauce
- ½ tsp. garlic powder

DIRECTIONS | **Ready in about:** 1 h 30 min

Heat the temperature of the air fryer to 356°F. Cut the wings into three sections (limb, middle joint and thigh). Dry them well with a paper towel. Mix the pepper, salt, garlic powder and cayenne pepper In a portable bowl by flow. Lightly coat the wings with powder. Spot the chicken on a wire rack and bake for 15 minutes, turning once every 7 minutes. Toss hot melted butter sauce on a plate to garnish the baked chicken when ready to serve.

119. Carrots and Chicken

INGREDIENTS | **Servings:** 2
- 2 carrots, sliced
- 4 stalks celery, sliced
- 1 onion, sliced
- 1 cup thyme
- 1 bay leaf
- 1 lb. chicken thighs
- 4 cups egg noodles
- 2 tbsp. lemon juice
- 3 cup chicken broth

DIRECTIONS | **Ready in about:** 12 min

Add chicken broth into the air fryer pot. Combine carrots, celery, onion, thyme, bay leaf, lemon juice and chicken thighs. Bake at 400°F for 10 minutes. Add the egg noodles and cook for another 10 minutes. When you are ready, help yourself and enjoy!

120. Cheese and Broccoli Chicken

INGREDIENTS | **Servings:** 2
- 2 tbsp. butter
- 1 lb. chicken breasts
- 3 cups broccoli
- 2 cups white rice, boiled
- 1 cup chicken stock
- 1 cup sour cream
- 1 tbsp. lemon juice
- 1 cup cheddar cheese, grated

DIRECTIONS | **Ready in about:** 20 min

Add butter into the air fryer pot. Mix the chicken breasts, broccoli, chicken broth, sour cream and lemon juice. Cook at 300°F for 15 minutes. Add the rice and cook for another 4 minutes. When it's ready, sprinkle with cheese to serve!

121. Chicken and Black Olives Sauce

INGREDIENTS | **Servings:** 2

- 2 tbsp. olive oil
- 1 chicken breast cut into 4 pieces
- 3 garlic cloves, minced

For the sauce:

- salt and black pepper to taste
- 1 cup black olives, pitted
- 2 tbsp. olive oil
- 1 tbsp. lemon juice
- ¼ cup parsley, chopped

DIRECTIONS | **Ready in about:** 18 min

In your food processor, combine the olives with salt, pepper, 2 tbsp. of olive oil, lemon juice and parsley, mix together and transfer to a bowl. Spice the chicken with salt and pepper, rub it with oil and garlic, put it in the preheated air fryer and bake at 370°F for 8 minutes. Divide the chicken between plates, top with olive sauce and serve.

122. Chicken and Bow Pasta

INGREDIENTS | **Servings:** 2

- 1 lb. bow tie pasta, boiled
- 1 lb. chicken breast, sliced
- 2 tbsp. Italian seasoning
- salt and pepper to taste
- 2 garlic cloves, minced
- 2 tbsp. red pepper flakes
- 2 cups ricotta cheese
- 1 cup basil leaves, chopped
- 1 onion, sliced

DIRECTIONS | **Ready in about:** 20 min

Add onion with salt and pepper into the air fryer pot. Mix the pasta, chicken, onion, the garlic, the flake pepper and ricotta. Cook at 300°F for 15 minutes. When finished, pour in the Italian vinaigrette. Serve garnished with basil.

123. Chicken and Capers

INGREDIENTS | **Servings:** 2

- 3 tbsp. capers
- 4 chicken thighs
- 4 garlic cloves, minced
- salt and black pepper to taste
- 3 tbsp. butter, melted
- ½ cup chicken stock
- 4 green onions, chopped
- 1 lemon, sliced

DIRECTIONS | **Ready in about:** 30 min

Brush the chicken with butter, sprinkle with salt and pepper to taste, put them in a pan suitable for your air fryer. Also add capers, garlic, chicken broth and lemon pieces, mix with the layer, put in the air-fryer and cook at 370°F for 20 minutes, stirring halfway cooking. Sprinkle with green onions, divide between plates and serve.

124. Chicken and Chestnuts Mix

INGREDIENTS | **Servings:** 2

- 1 small yellow onion, chopped
- ½ pound chicken pieces
- 2 tsp. garlic, minced
- 1 pinch of allspice, ground
- 1 pinch of ginger, grated
- 4 tbsp. water chestnuts
- 2 tortillas for serving
- 2 tbsp. chicken stock
- 2 tbsp. soy sauce
- 2 tbsp. balsamic vinegar

DIRECTIONS | **Ready in about:** 22 min

In a pan suitable for your air fryer, mix the chicken meat with the onion, garlic, ginger, allspice, chestnuts, soy sauce, broth and vinegar, stir, transfer to your air fryer and bake at 360°F for 12 minutes. Divide everything between plates and serve.

125. Chicken and Spinach Salad

INGREDIENTS | **Servings:** 2

- 2 chicken breasts, skinless and boneless
- 2 tsp. parsley, dried
- ½ tsp. onion powder
- ½ cup lemon juice
- 2 tsp. sweet paprika
- salt and black pepper to taste
- 8 strawberries, sliced
- 5 cups baby spinach
- 1 small red onion, sliced
- 1 tbsp. tarragon, chopped
- 1 avocado, pitted, peeled and chopped
- 2 tbsp. balsamic vinegar
- ¼ cup olive oil

DIRECTIONS | **Ready in about:** 22 min

Put the chicken in a portable bowl, add the lemon juice, parsley, onion powder and paprika and mix. Transfer it to your air fryer and cook at 360°F for 12 minutes. In a portable bowl, combine the spinach, onion, strawberries and avocado and toss. In another portable bowl, combine the oil with the vinegar, salt, pepper and tarragon, beat well, add to the salad and mix. Divide the chicken between plates, add the spinach salad on the side and serve.

126. Chicken Breast with Marsala

INGREDIENTS | **Servings:** 2

- 1 lb. chicken breast, sliced
- 1 cup Marsala wine
- 1 tbsp. cumin powder
- salt and pepper to taste
- 2 tbsp. butter
- 1 cup parsley leaves, chopped

DIRECTIONS | **Ready in about:** 25 min

Add chicken breast and butter into the air fryer. Mix Marsala, cumin powder, butter with salt and pepper. Cook at 300°F for 20 minutes. Garnish with the parsley to serve.

127. Chicken Kabobs

INGREDIENTS | **Servings:** 2

- 1/3 cup honey
- 2 chicken breasts
- 1/3 cup soy sauce
- 6 mushrooms
- sesame seeds
- 1 each for green, red and yellow bell pepper
- salt to taste
- cooking spray

DIRECTIONS | **Ready in about:** 30 min

Cut the chicken breast into cubes. Spray the cubes with cooking spray and season with salt and pepper. Transfer to a bowl and toss the chicken with the honey, soy sauce and sesame seeds. Cut the mushrooms in half. Preheat the air fryer to 340°F. Include the chicken, peppers and mushrooms to the kebab skewers (metal skewers work best in an air fryer) alternating until the skewers are full. Cook for 20 minutes, turning the skewers in half.

128. Chicken Parmesan Cutlets

INGREDIENTS | **Servings:** 2

- 2 tbsp. parmesan cheese, grated
- 1 cup Panko breadcrumbs
- ¼ tsp. garlic powder
- 1 egg, whisked
- 1 cup white flour
- ¾ pound skinless, boneless chicken cutlets
- ½ cup mozzarella, grated
- 1½ tbsp. basil, chopped
- salt and pepper, to taste
- 1 cup tomato sauce

DIRECTIONS | **Ready in about:** 25 min

In a portable bowl, combine the garlic powder and Parmesan cheese and mix. Put the flour in a second bowl. Put the egg in a third and beat. Season the chicken with salt and pepper. Dip in the flour, then in the egg mixture. Finally, garnish with panko. Cook the chicken pieces in the air fryer at 360°F for 3 minutes on each side. Transfer the chicken to a baking sheet. Add the tomato sauce and garnish with the mozzarella. Bake in an air fryer at 375°F for 7 minutes. Divide among plates, sprinkle with basil and serve.

129. Chicken Tenders

INGREDIENTS | **Servings:** 2

- 1 lb. chicken tenders
- 2 garlic cloves, minced
- 2 tbsp. paprika
- 2 tbsp. oregano powder
- salt and pepper to taste
- 2 tbsp. oil
- 1 onion, chopped
- 2 cups peas (frozen)
- 1 cup flour (all-purpose)
- 1 cup chicken stock
- 1 egg

DIRECTIONS | **Ready in about:** 15 min

Add oil into the air fryer pot. Mix chicken fillets, garlic, paprika, oregano, onion, peas, flour and chicken broth. Add the egg with salt and pepper. Cook at 300°F for 10 minutes. Serve and enjoy!

130. Chicken Thighs with Stock

INGREDIENTS | **Servings:** 2

- 1 lb. chicken thighs
- salt and pepper to taste
- 3 tbsp. oil
- 1 tbsp. butter
- 2 tbsp. flour
- 1 cup chicken stock
- 2 tbsp. lemon juice
- bread for serving

DIRECTIONS | **Ready in about:** 22 min

Add oil into the air fryer pot. Mix the chicken thighs, butter, flour, chicken broth, the juice of lemon with salt and pepper. Cook at 300°F for 20 minutes. Serve with bread to taste!

131. Chicken Wings

INGREDIENTS | **Servings:** 2

- oil in spay
- 10 chicken wings
- 1 tbsp. soy sauce
- 2 tbsp. honey
- ½ tbsp. cornstarch
- 1 tbsp. ground fresh chili paste
- ½ tsp. chopped fresh ginger
- 1 tbsp. minced garlic
- 1 tbsp. lime sumo
- 2 tbsp. chives
- ½ tbsp. salt

DIRECTIONS | **Ready in about:** 35 min

Pat the chicken dry with a tea towel. Coat chicken with cooking spray. Place the chicken in the electric hot-air fryer, spreading the wings out towards the edge so they don't overlap. Bake at 400°F until it that the crispy skin for about 25 min. Flip them half the time. Combine the soy sauce with the cornstarch in a saucepan. Add honey, chili paste, garlic, ginger, and lime sumo. Cook over low heat until boiling and thickening. Place the chicken in a portable bowl, add the sauce and coat all the chicken. Sprinkle with chives.

132. Chicken Wings with Hot Sauce

INGREDIENTS | **Servings:** 2

- 2 cups flour (all-purpose)
- 2 tbsp. Cayenne powder
- 2 tbsp. oil
- 1 lb. chicken wings
- 1 tbsp. butter
- salt to taste
- 1 tbsp. lemon juice
- 1 tbsp. hot sauce

DIRECTIONS | **Ready in about:** 15 min

Add oil into the air fryer pot. Combine the cayenne powder, flour, salt, butter and lemon juice in the bowl. Dip the chicken wings and put them in the pan. Cook at 400°F for 10 minutes. Add the hot sauce. When it's ready, serve and enjoy!

133. Chicken with Apple

INGREDIENTS | **Servings:** 2

- 1 tbsp. fresh ginger, finely grated
- 1 shallot, thinly sliced
- 1 tsp. fresh thyme, minced
- 2 tbsp. maple syrup
- 1 large apple, cored and cubed
- ½ cup apple cider
- salt and ground black pepper, as required
- 2 (4 ounces) boneless, skinless chicken thighs, sliced into chunks

DIRECTIONS | **Ready in about:** 40 min

In a portable bowl, combine the shallot, ginger, thyme, apple cider, maple syrup, salt and black pepper. Add the chicken pieces and toss generously with the marinade. Marinate in the refrigerator for 6-8 hours. Set the air-fryer temperature to 390°F. Grease a fryer basket. Place the chicken pieces and the diced apple in the air fryer basket. Air fry for about 20 minutes, flipping once halfway. Remove from the fryer and transfer the chicken mixture to a serving plate. Serve hot.

134. Chicken with Black Beans

INGREDIENTS | **Servings:** 2

- 1 lb. chicken breasts, pieces
- salt and pepper to taste
- 2 tbsp. butter
- 1 cup parsley leaves, chopped
- 2 cups black beans
- 1 tomato, chopped

DIRECTIONS | **Ready in about:** 18 min

Add butter into the air fryer pot. Toss black beans, tomatoes, parsley, chicken with salt and pepper. Cook at 300°F for 15 minutes. When it's ready, help yourself and enjoy!

135. Chicken with Buttermilk

INGREDIENTS | **Servings:** 2

- 2 tbsp. lemon zest
- 1 tbsp. brown sugar
- 1 cup buttermilk
- 1 lb. chicken drumsticks
- salt and pepper to taste
- 2 tbsp. thyme
- 1 cup mayonnaise
- 2 tbsp. oil
- 2 tbsp. Cayenne powder

DIRECTIONS | **Ready in about:** 20 min

Add oil into the air fryer pot. Mix lemon zest, brown sugar, buttermilk, chicken drumsticks, thyme, cayenne pepper powder with salt and pepper. Cook at 300°F for 15 minutes. When it's ready, serve it with mayonnaise and enjoy your meal!

136. Chicken with Garlic

INGREDIENTS | **Servings:** 2

- 1 lb. roasted chicken, sliced
- salt and pepper to taste
- 1 tbsp. lemon juice
- 2 tbsp. butter
- 1 onion, chopped
- 2 carrots, chopped
- 2 garlic cloves, minced

DIRECTIONS | **Ready in about:** 17 min

Add roasted chicken into the air fryer pot. Combine the lemon juice, butter, onion, carrots, garlic with salt and pepper. Bake at 300°F for 15 minutes. Serve and enjoy!

137. Chicken with Lemon Juice

INGREDIENTS | **Servings:** 2

- 1 tbsp. thyme
- salt and pepper to taste
- 2 tbsp. oil
- 1 yellow onion, chopped
- 1 cup olives, halves
- 1 lb. chicken, shredded
- 1 cup white wine
- 1 tbsp. lemon juice
- 2 garlic cloves, minced

DIRECTIONS | **Ready in about:** 20 min

Add oil into the air fryer pot. Mix the onion, thyme, olives, chicken. White wine, lemon juice and garlic. Cook at 300°F for 15 minutes. When it's ready, help yourself and enjoy!

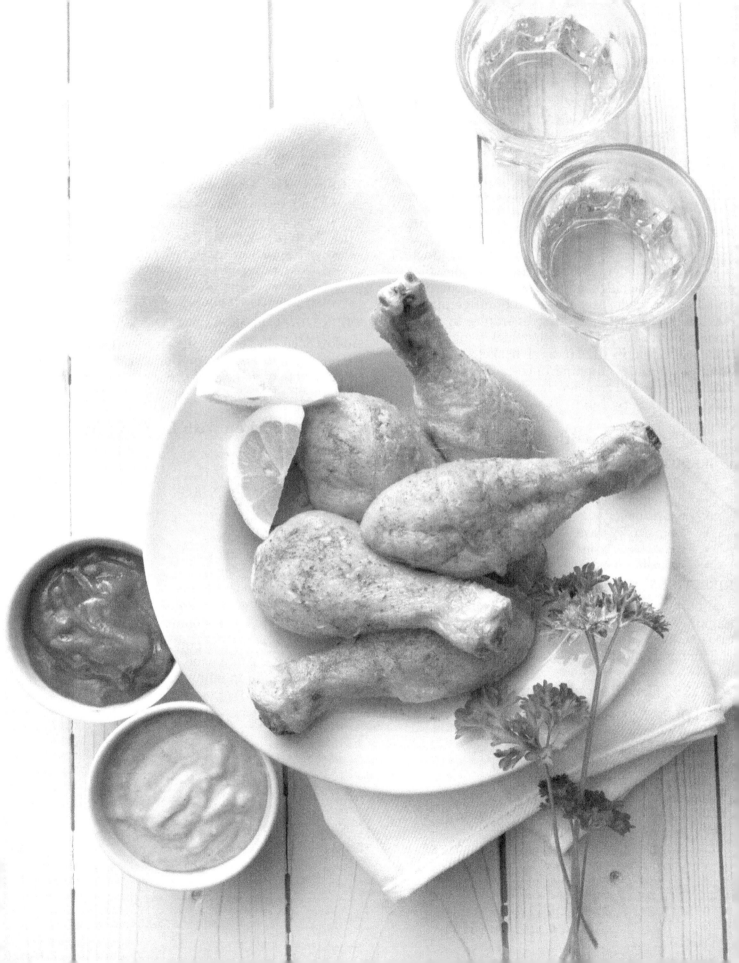

138. Chicken with Lemon Zest

INGREDIENTS | Servings: 2

- 2 cups breadcrumbs
- 2 tbsp. lemon zest
- 1 tbsp. thyme
- salt and pepper to taste
- 2 cups flour (all-purpose)
- 1 lb. chicken breast, sliced
- 2 tbsp. oil

DIRECTIONS | Ready in about: 20 min

Add the flour and lemon zest to the bowl. Mix the thyme, breadcrumbs with salt and pepper. Coat the chicken with oil and dip in the mixture. Add the chicken to the air fryer. Cook at 300°F for 15 minutes. When it's ready, serve and enjoy your meal.

139. Chicken with Mushrooms

INGREDIENTS | Servings: 2

- 2 tbsp. oil
- 2 tbsp. soy sauce
- 1 lb. chicken thighs, sliced
- 2 garlic cloves, minced
- 2 jalapeno peppers, chopped
- 2 cups mushrooms, chopped
- 2 cups cabbage, chopped
- 3 cup chicken stock
- salt and pepper to taste
- 3 cups noodles
- cilantro and peanuts for garnishing

DIRECTIONS | Ready in about: 22 min

Add oil into the air fryer pot. Combine soy sauce, chicken thighs, garlic, jalapeño peppers, mushrooms et al. Add the chicken broth, salted and peppered noodles. Cook at 300°F for 20 minutes. When finished, serve with the cilantro and peanut vinaigrette.

140. Chicken with Potatoes

INGREDIENTS | Servings: 2

- 2 red potatoes, cubed
- 1 tbsp. cumin seeds
- 2 tbsp. oil
- 2 garlic cloves, minced
- 1 lb. chicken, cubed
- 2 tbsp. red pepper flakes
- salt and pepper to taste
- cilantro leaves, chopped to garnish

DIRECTIONS | Ready in about: 18 min

Add oil into the air fryer pot. Mix red potatoes, cumin seeds, garlic, chicken, the flakes of chili red with salt and pepper. Cook at 300°F for 15 minutes. When finished, garnish with cilantro to serve!

141. Chicken with Scallions

INGREDIENTS | Servings: 2

- 1 lb. chicken, diced
- 2 cups scallions, chopped
- 1 tbsp. dill
- 1 tbsp. lemon juice
- salt and pepper to taste
- parsley, chopped, to garnish

DIRECTIONS | Ready in about: 20 min

Add chicken into the air fryer pot. Mix the scallions, dill, lemon juice, parsley with salt and pepper. Cook at 300°F for 15 minutes. Serve and enjoy!

142. Chicken with Spices

INGREDIENTS | Servings: 2

- 2 tbsp. oil
- 2 garlic cloves, minced
- 2 tbsp. lemon juice
- 2 tbsp. oregano
- salt and pepper to taste
- 1 lb. chicken breast
- cheese, grated, to garnish

DIRECTIONS | Ready in about: 20 min

Add oil into the air fryer pot. Combine the garlic cloves, lemon juice, oregano, chicken breast with salt and pepper. Cook at 400°F for 15 minutes. When it's ready, top the cheese for serving!

143. Chicken Garlic Turkey

INGREDIENTS | **Servings:** 2

- 1 onion, sliced
- 2 tomatoes, sliced
- 2 garlic cloves, minced
- 2 tbsp. chili garlic sauce
- 1 tbsp. sugar
- 1 lb. turkey, minced
- 2 tbsp. ginger, grated
- 3 tbsp. oil
- 2 cups scallions, chopped

DIRECTIONS | **Ready in about:** 20 min

Add oil into the air fryer pot. Combine the onion, tomatoes, garlic, hot garlic sauce, sugar, turkey, ginger and chives. Cook at 300°F for 15 minutes. When it's ready, serve!

144. Chinese Duck Legs

INGREDIENTS | **Servings:** 2

- 2 dried chilies, chopped
- 2 duck legs
- 1 tbsp. olive oil
- 1 bunch spring onions, chopped
- 2 stars anise
- 1 tbsp. soy sauce
- 1 tbsp. oyster sauce
- 1 tsp. sesame oil
- 1 tbsp. rice wine
- 14 ounces water
- 4 ginger slices

DIRECTIONS | **Ready in about:** 47 min

Over medium heat, bring the oven and add pepper, star anise, the oil sesame, rice wine, ginger, oyster sauce, soy sauce and water, stir and cook for 6 minutes. Add the chives and feet duck, stir to coat the transfer to an appropriate air fryer and cook at 370°F for 30 minutes. Divide into plates and serve.

145. Creamy Stock

INGREDIENTS | **Servings:** 2

- 1 green bell pepper, chopped
- 1 lb. chicken, shredded
- 1 cup cabbage
- 3 cup cream of chicken stock
- 1 cup buttermilk
- salt and pepper to taste

DIRECTIONS | **Ready in about:** 20 min

Add buttermilk into the air fryer pot. Mix green pepper, chicken, cabbage, cream broth with salt and pepper. Cook at 300°F for 15 minutes. When it's ready, help yourself and enjoy!

146. Crispy Chicken Wings

INGREDIENTS | **Servings:** 2

- 1 onion, finely chopped
- 2 lemongrass stalk, white portion, minced
- 1 tbsp. soy sauce
- salt and ground white pepper, as required
- ½ cup cornstarch
- 1½ tbsp. honey
- 1 pound chicken wings, rinsed and trimmed

DIRECTIONS | **Ready in about:** 45 min

In a portable bowl, combine the lemongrass, onion, soy sauce, honey, salt and white pepper. Add the wings and cover generously with the marinade. Cover and refrigerate to marinate overnight. Set the temperature of the fryer to 355°F. Grease a basket of the air fryer. Take off the chicken wing from the marinade and cover with the cornstarch. Place the chicken wings in the prepared air fryer basket in a single layer. Air fry for about 25 minutes, turning them in half at once. Remove from the air fryer and transfer the chicken wings to a serving plate. Serve hot.

147. Duck and Cherries

INGREDIENTS | Servings: 2

- ¼ cup honey
- ½ cup of sugar
- 1/3 cup balsamic vinegar
- 1 tbsp. ginger, grated
- 1 tsp. garlic, minced
- 1 tsp. cumin, ground
- ½ tsp. cinnamon powder
- salt and black pepper to taste
- ½ tsp. clove, ground
- 4 sage leaves, chopped
- 2 cups rhubarb, sliced
- 1 jalapeno, chopped
- ½ cup yellow onion, chopped
- 4 duck breasts, boneless, skin on and scored
- 2 cups cherries, pitted

DIRECTIONS | Ready in about: 30 min

Spice the duck breast with salt and pepper, place in the air fryer and cook at 350°F for 5 minutes per side. Meanwhile, heat a skillet over medium heat, add the sugar, honey, vinegar, garlic, ginger, cumin, cloves, cinnamon, sage, jalapeno, rhubarb, onion and cherries, stir, bring to a boil and cook for 10 minutes. Add the duck breasts, mix well, divide everything into plates and serve.

148. Duck and Plum Sauce

INGREDIENTS | Servings: 2

- 1 tbsp. butter, melted
- 2 duck breasts
- 1 star anise
- 1 shallot, chopped
- 1 tbsp. olive oil
- 9 ounces red plumps, stoned, cut into small wedges
- 2 tbsp. red wine
- 2 tbsp. sugar
- 1 cup beef stock

DIRECTIONS | Ready in about: 45 min

Heat a pan with olive oil over medium heat, add the shallot, stir and cook for 5 minutes, add the sugar and the prunes, stir and cook until the sugar dissolves. Add the broth and wine, mix, cook for 15 minutes, remove from the heat and keep warm for now. Slice the duck breasts, season with salt and pepper, rub the butter melted, transfer to a plate heat resistant suitable for air fryer, add the sauce with star anise and plum placed in the fryer air and cook at 360°F for 12 minutes. Divide everything between plates and serve.

149. Duck with Balsamic Vinegar

INGREDIENTS | Servings: 2

- 1 cup thyme
- 2 garlic cloves, minced
- 1 lb. frozen duck, slices
- 2 shallots, minced
- 2 tbsp. balsamic vinegar
- 2 cups corn kernels

DIRECTIONS | Ready in about: 23 min

Add garlic into the air fryer pot. Mix thyme, duck, shallot, corn grains and the vinegar balsamic. Cook at 400°F for 20 minutes. Serve and enjoy!

150. Honey Duck Breast

INGREDIENTS | Servings: 2

- 1 tsp. honey
- 1 tsp. tomato paste
- ½ tsp. apple vinegar
- 1 smoked duck breast, halved
- 1 tbsp. mustard

DIRECTIONS | Ready in about: 32 min

In a portable bowl, mix the honey with the tomato paste, mustard and vinegar, beat well, add the pieces of duck breast, stir to coat them well, transfer to the air fryer and cook at 370°F for 15 minutes. Remove the duck breast from the fryer, add it to the honey mixture, mix again, return to the air fryer and boil at 370°F for 6 minutes. Divide among plates and serve with a salad garnish.

151. Jalapeno and Avocado Chicken

INGREDIENTS | Servings: 2

- 2 tbsp. oil
- 1 onion, chopped
- 1 cup jalapenos, chopped
- 1 lb. chicken, sliced
- 2 cups red kidney beans
- 2 avocados, chopped
- 2 cilantro leaves, chopped, to garnish

DIRECTIONS | Ready in about: 18 min

Add oil into the air fryer pot. Stir in onion, jalapeño peppers, chicken, kidney beans and avocado. Bake at 300°F for 15 minutes. When finished, garnish with cilantro to serve!

152. Marinated Duck Breasts

INGREDIENTS | **Servings:** 2

- 1 cup white wine
- 2 duck breasts
- ¼ cup of soy sauce
- 6 tarragon springs
- 2 garlic cloves, minced
- 1 tbsp. butter
- salt and black pepper to taste
- ¼ cup sherry wine

DIRECTIONS | **Ready in about:** 24 h 20 min

In a portable bowl, mix the duck breasts with the white wine, soy sauce, garlic, tarragon, salt and pepper, mix them together and refrigerate for 1 day. Transfer the duck breast to your air fryer preheated to 350°F and cook for 10 minutes, turning halfway. Meanwhile, pour the marinade into a pan, heat over medium heat, add the butter and sherry, mix, bring to a boil, cook for 5 minutes and remove from the heat. Divide the duck breasts between plates, drizzle with the sauce and serve.

153. Mexican Chicken Breast

INGREDIENTS | **Servings:** 2

- ½ tbsp. olive oil
- 8 ounces salsa verde
- salt and black pepper, to taste
- ¾ cup Monetary Jack cheese, grated
- ½ tsp. garlic powder
- ½ pound boneless, skinless chicken breast
- 2 tbsp. cilantro, chopped

DIRECTIONS | **Ready in about:** 30 min

Pour the salsa verde into a baking dish. Season the chicken with salt, pepper, garlic powder and brush with olive oil. Place over the salsa verde. Spot the pan in the air fryer and cook at 380°F for 20 minutes. Sprinkle with cheese and cook for another 2 minutes.

154. Roasted Chicken with Mayo

INGREDIENTS | **Servings:** 2

- 1 lb. roasted chicken
- 1 cup raisins
- 2 tbsp. oil
- 1 cup almonds, sliced
- 2 scallions, chopped
- 1 cup mayonnaise
- 3 cup Greek yogurt
- 2 tbsp. curry powder
- 3 tsp. sugar
- salt and pepper to taste
- cilantro leaves for garnishing

DIRECTIONS | **Ready in about:** 13 min

Add oil into the air fryer pot. Combine the roast chicken, raisins, almonds, shallots, curry powder, sugar with salt and pepper. Cook at 300°F for 10 minutes. Combine mayonnaise and green yogurt in the bowl. When the chicken is ready, decorate the cilantro leaves. Serve with the mayonnaise mixture to enjoy!

155. Tomato Sauce Chicken

INGREDIENTS | **Servings:** 2

- 1 tbsp. garlic powder
- 1 tbsp. dried cumin
- 1 tbsp. salt and pepper to taste
- 1 lb. chicken boneless, sliced
- 2 garlic cloves, minced
- 2 cups rice, boiled
- 2 cups tomato sauce
- 1 red bell pepper, sliced
- 1 onion, sliced

DIRECTIONS | **Ready in about:** 18 min

Add garlic and cumin into the air fryer pot. Combine chicken, tomato sauce, red pepper, onion with salt and pepper. Cook at 300°F for 15 minutes. Add the rice and cook for another 4 minutes. Serve and enjoy!

156. White Beans with Chicken

INGREDIENTS | Servings: 2

- 2 cans white beans
- 1 jalapeno pepper, minced
- 2 Poblano peppers, chopped
- 1 onion, chopped
- 3 tbsp. oil
- 2 garlic cloves, minced
- salt and pepper to taste
- 1 tbsp. coriander powder
- 2 cups chicken broth
- 1 lb. chicken, sliced
- 1 tbsp. chili powder
- cilantro leaves for garnishing
- tortilla chips, for topping

DIRECTIONS | Ready in about: 30 min

Add oil into the air fryer pot. Combine the garlic, cilantro powder, chili powder, onion, poblano peppers, jalapeno peppers, chicken and chicken broth. Cook at 300°F for 15 minutes. Add the white beans. Cook for another 10 minutes. When cooked, garnish with cilantro and tortilla chips for serving.

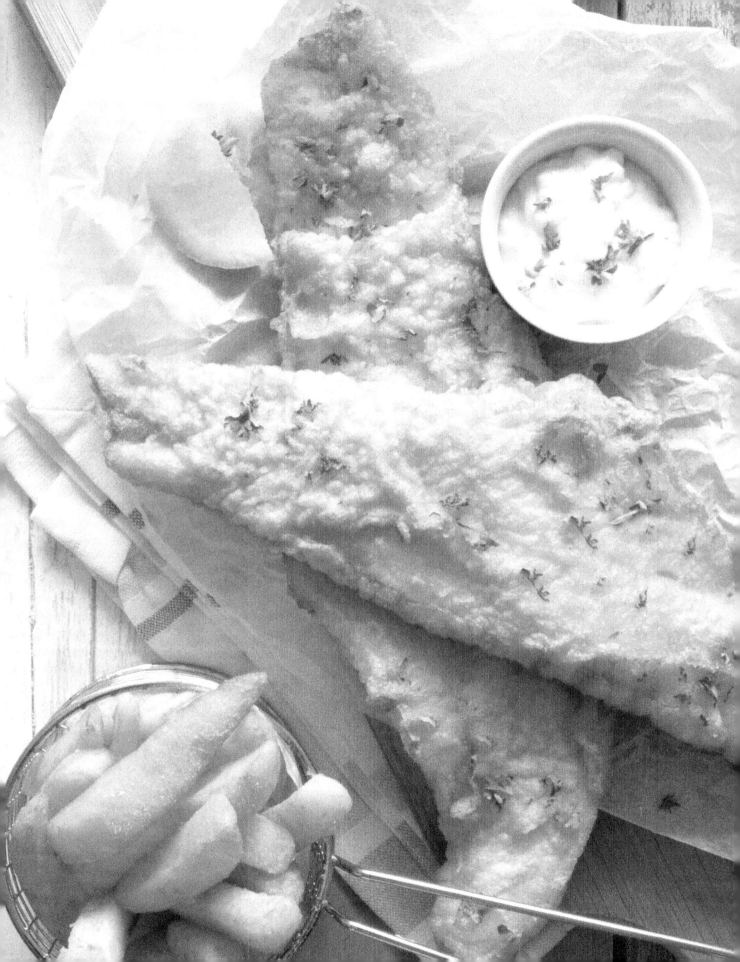

FISH & SEAFOOD

157. Almond Pesto Salmon

INGREDIENTS | Servings: 2
- ¼ cup sliced almonds, roughly chopped
- 2 tbsp. unsalted butter, melted
- ¼ cup pesto
- 2 salmon fillets (about 4 ounces each)

DIRECTIONS | Ready in about: 20 min

In a portable small bowl, combine the pesto and almonds. Set besides. In a 6' round baking dish, spot the fillets. Brush each fillet with butter and put half of the pesto mixture on each fillet. Spot the dish in the basket of the air fryer. Set the temperature to 390°F and set the timer for 12 minutes the salmon flakes easily when fully cooked and reaches an internal temperature of at least 145°F. Serve hot.

158. Amazing Salmon Fillets

INGREDIENTS | Servings: 2
- 1 tbsp. Italian seasoning
- 2 (¾-inch thick) salmon fillets
- 1 tbsp. fresh lemon juice

DIRECTIONS | Ready in about: 12 min

Preheat the air fryer to 355°F and grease an Air fryer grill pan. Rub uniformly salmon with Italian dressing and transfer to the Air fryer grill pan, skin side up. Cook for about 7 minutes and squeeze the lemon juice to serve.

159. Asian Salmon

INGREDIENTS | Servings: 2
- 6 tbsp. light soy sauce
- 2 medium salmon fillets
- 3 tsp. mirin
- 6 tbsp. honey
- 1 tsp. water

DIRECTIONS | Ready in about: 1 h 15 min

In a portable bowl, mix the soy sauce with the honey, water and mirin, beat well, add the salmon, rub well and set aside in the refrigerator for 1 hour. Transfer the salmon to your air fryer and cook at 360°F for 15 minutes, flipping after 7 minutes. Meanwhile, put the soy marinade in a pan, heat over medium heat, beat well, cook 2 minutes and remove from heat. Divide the salmon among plates, sprinkle with marinade and serve.!

160. Black Beans with Ham and Salmon

INGREDIENTS | Servings: 2
- 2 lb. ham hock
- 1 lb. salmon, chopped
- 1 onion, chopped
- 2 garlic cloves, minced
- 2 cups black beans
- 2 bay leaves
- 2 tbsp. oregano powder

DIRECTIONS | Ready in about: 13 min

Add onion and bay leaves into the air fryer pot. Combine the shank, garlic, black beans and oregano powder. Bake at 300°F for 9 minutes. When finished, serve and enjoy!

161. Black Beans with Mackerel

INGREDIENTS | **Servings:** 2

- 4 cups black beans
- 3 onions, chopped
- 2 tbsp. olive oil
- salt to taste
- 1 lb. mackerel fillets
- 1 tbsp. oregano
- 1 tbsp. chili powder
- ½ cup green chilies
- cilantro leaves to garnish

DIRECTIONS | **Ready in about:** 15 min

Add oil into the air fryer pot. Toss the onions, mackerel fillets, salt, oregano, green peppers and chili powder with the black beans. Cook at 300°F for 10 minutes. When finished, serve and enjoy the food.

162. Cajun Salmon

INGREDIENTS | **Servings:** 2

- 2 tbsp. unsalted butter, melted
- 2 (4 ounces) salmon fillets, skin removed
- ⅛ tsp. ground cayenne pepper
- ¼ tsp. ground black pepper
- 1 tsp. paprika
- ½ tsp. garlic powder

DIRECTIONS | **Ready in about:** 15 min

Butter each fillet. Mix the other ingredients in a little bowl then rub onto fish. Place the steaks in the fryer basket. Set the temperature to 390°F and set the timer for 7 minutes. Serve immediately. serve.

163. Celery and Salmon Fillets

INGREDIENTS | **Servings:** 2

- 1 lb. salmon fillets
- 3 stalks chopped celery
- 2 garlic cloves
- 2 onion, chopped
- salt and pepper to taste
- 2 cups green onion, chopped

DIRECTIONS | **Ready in about:** 20 min

Add salmon fillets into the air fryer pot. Combine celery, garlic, salt and pepper, the onion and the onion green. Cook at 300°F for 15 minutes. When it's ready, help yourself and enjoy!

164. Chickpeas and Shrimp

INGREDIENTS | **Servings:** 2

- 2 cups chickpeas
- 1 lb. shrimps
- 2 cups vegetable broth
- 2 cups red lentils
- 1 tbsp. cumin powder
- 1 tbsp. coriander powder
- 2 tbsp. tomato paste
- 1 tbsp. ginger, minced
- 1 tbsp. lime juice
- chopped cilantro for garnishing

DIRECTIONS | **Ready in about:** 20 min

Add ginger into the air fryer pot. Combine the shrimp, chickpeas, vegetable broth and lime juice. Cook at 300°F for 4 minutes. Now add the cumin, coriander, red lentils and tomato paste. Cook for another 10 minutes. When ready, garnish with cilantro and serve.

165. Chickpeas with Crab

INGREDIENTS | **Servings:** 2

- 1 tbsp. curry powder
- 1 tbsp. black pepper
- 1 tbsp. oil
- salt to taste
- 1 tbsp. mustard seeds
- 2 cloves garlic, minced
- 3 cups red kidney beans
- 3 cups chickpeas
- 1 lb. crabmeat
- 1 cup water

DIRECTIONS | **Ready in about:** 18 min

Add oil to the air fryer pot. Add the chickpeas and mix well. Add the curry powder, mustard seeds, chickpeas, beans, garlic, water and black pepper. Add the crab meat. Cook at 300°F for 20 minutes. Serve and enjoy!

166. Cilantro Lime Baked Salmon

INGREDIENTS | Servings: 2

- 1 tbsp. salted butter, melted
- 2 (3 ounces) salmon fillets, skin removed
- 1 tsp. chili powder
- 2 tbsp. chopped cilantro
- ¼ cup sliced pickled jalapeños
- ½ tsp. finely minced garlic
- ½ medium lime, juiced

DIRECTIONS | Ready in about: 22 min

Place the salmon fillets in a 6-inch round skillet. Brush each with butter and sprinkle with chili powder and garlic. Place the jalapeno slices on top and around the salmon. Pour half of the lime juice over the salmon and cover with a sheet of aluminum. Spot the pan in the air fryer basket. Adjust the temperature to 370°F and set timer f or 12 minutes. When cooked, the salmon should flake easily with a fork and reach a core temperature of at least 145°F. To serve, drizzle with remaining lemon juice and garnish with cilantro.

167. Coconut Shrimp

INGREDIENTS | Servings: 2

- 2 tbsp. salted butter, melted
- ¼ cup unsweetened shredded coconut
- 8 ounces medium shelled and deveined shrimp
- ½ tsp. Old Bay seasoning
- 1 tsp. sweet paprika
- 1 tsp. mustard powder
- salt and black pepper to taste
- 6 chicken breasts, skinless and boneless
- 1 tsp. garlic powder

DIRECTIONS | Ready in about: 12 min

In an enormous bowl, toss the shrimp with the butter and Old Bay seasoning. Put the grated coconut in the bowl. Cover each piece of shrimp with coconut and place in the air fryer basket. Set the air-fryer temperature to 400°F and set the timer for 6 minutes. Turn the shrimp turn halfway through the cooking period. Serve immediately.

168. Cod Fillets with Fennel and Grapes Salad

INGREDIENTS | Servings: 2

- 1 tbsp. olive oil
- 2 black cod fillets, boneless
- salt and black pepper to taste
- ½ cup pecans
- 1 cup grapes, halved
- 1 fennel bulb, thinly sliced

DIRECTIONS | Ready in about: 25 min

Pour half the oil over the fish fillets, season with salt and pepper, rub well, put the fillets in the air-fryer basket, cook for approximately 10 minutes at 400°F and transfer to a plate. In a bowl, toss the nuts with the raisins, fennel, remaining oil, salt and pepper, toss to coat, add to a pan that fits your air fryer and cook at 400°F for 5 minutes. Divide the cod into plates, add the fennel and mixed grapes on the side and serve.

169. Cod Fillets with Squash

INGREDIENTS | Servings: 2

- 1 lb. cod fillets
- 2 cups squash, chopped
- salt to taste
- 2 tbsp. tomato sauce
- 2 cups beans
- 1 tbsp. cumin powder

DIRECTIONS | Ready in about: 18 min

Add cod fillets into the air fryer pot. Combine the pumpkin, tomato sauce, beans and cumin powder. Add the salt. Cook at 300°F for 10 minutes. When it's ready, serve and enjoy!

170. Cod Steaks with Plum Sauce

INGREDIENTS | **Servings:** 2

- salt and black pepper to taste
- 2 big cod steaks
- ½ tsp. garlic powder
- ¼ tsp. turmeric powder
- cooking spray
- ½ tsp. ginger powder
- 1 tbsp. plum sauce

DIRECTIONS | **Ready in about:** 30 min

Spice the cod fillets with salt and pepper, sprinkle with cooking oil, add garlic powder, ginger powder and turmeric powder and rub well. Place the cod fillets in the air fryer and cook at 360°F for 15 minutes, turning after 7 minutes. Heat a pan over medium heat, add the plum sauce, mix and cook for 2 minutes. Divide the cod fillets between plates, sprinkle with plum sauce and serve.

171. Cod with Celery Stalk

INGREDIENTS | **Servings:** 2

- 2 carrots, sliced
- 2 cups vegetable broth
- 1 lb. cod, cubed
- salt to taste
- 4 cups cauliflower florets
- 2 tbsp. garlic, minced
- 2 tbsp. thyme, dried
- 4 celery stalks
- 1 tbsp. cornstarch

DIRECTIONS | **Ready in about:** 16 min

Add vegetable broth into the air fryer pot. Add the celery stalks, cornstarch, cod, thyme, garlic, cauliflower, salt and carrots. Cook at 300°F for 15 minutes. When it's ready, help yourself and enjoy!

172. Cod with Pearl Onions

INGREDIENTS | **Servings:** 2

- 2 medium cod fillets
- 14 ounces pearl onions
- 1 tbsp. parsley, dried
- 8 ounces mushrooms, sliced
- black pepper to taste
- 1 tsp. thyme, dried

DIRECTIONS | **Ready in about:** 25 min

Place the fish in a heat-resistant dish suitable for your air fryer, add the onion, parsley, mushrooms, thyme and black pepper, mix well, put in an air fryer and cook at 350°F and leave cook for 15 minutes. Divide everything between plates and serve.

173. Creamy Salmon

INGREDIENTS | **Servings:** 2

- 1 tbsp. chopped dill
- 1 tbsp. olive oil
- 3 tbsp. sour cream
- 2 ounces plain yogurt
- 6 pieces salmon

DIRECTIONS | **Ready in about:** 30 min

Heat the air fryer and wait for it to reach 285°F. Shake the salt over the salmon and add it to the air fryer basket along with the olive oil to sauté for 10 minutes. Stir in yogurt, salt and dill. Serve the salmon with the sauce with your favorite sides.

174. Crumbled Fish

INGREDIENTS | **Servings:** 2

- ½ cup breadcrumbs
- 4 tbsp. vegetable oil
- 1 egg
- 4 fish fillets
- 1 lemon

DIRECTIONS | **Ready in about:** 22 min

Heat the air fryer to 356°F. Stir in oil and breadcrumbs until crumbly. Steep the fish in the egg, then the breadcrumb mixture. Place the fish in the cooker and air fry for 12 minutes. Garnish with lemon.

175. Flavored Air Fried Salmon

INGREDIENTS | Servings: 2

- 2 tbsp. lemon juice
- 2 salmon fillets
- salt and black pepper to taste
- 2 tbsp. olive oil
- 1/3 cup water
- ½ tsp. garlic powder
- 1/3 cup soy sauce
- 1/3 cup brown sugar
- 3 scallions, chopped

DIRECTIONS | Ready in about: 1 h 18 min

In a portable bowl mix the sugar with the water, soy sauce, garlic powder, salt, pepper, oil and lemon juice, beat well, add the salmon fillets, mix until than the cream and let stand in the refrigerator for 1 hour. Transfer the salmon fillets to the basket of the air fryer and bake at 360°F for 8 minutes flipping them halfway. Divide the salmon between plates, sprinkle with shallots and serve immediately.

176. Foil-Packet Lobster Tail

INGREDIENTS | Servings: 2

- 2 tbsp. salted butter, melted
- 2 (6 ounces) lobster tails, halved
- ½ tsp. Old Bay seasoning
- 1 tsp. dried parsley
- juice of ½ medium lemon

DIRECTIONS | Ready in about: 30 min

Place the two tails halved on a sheet paper of aluminum. Drizzle with butter, Old Bay dressing and lemon juice. Seal the foil wrappers by completely covering the tails. Place in the fryer basket. Set the air-fryer temperature to 375°F and set the timer for 12 minutes. Once cooked, sprinkle with dried parsley and serve immediately.

177. Halibut and Sun-Dried Tomatoes Mix

INGREDIENTS | Servings: 2

- 2 garlic cloves, minced
- 2 medium halibut fillets
- 2 tsp. olive oil
- 6 sun-dried tomatoes, chopped
- salt and black pepper to taste
- 2 small red onions, sliced
- ½ tsp. red pepper flakes, crushed
- 9 black olives, pitted and sliced
- 1 fennel bulb, sliced
- 4 rosemary springs, chopped

DIRECTIONS | Ready in about: 20 min

Season the fish with salt, pepper, rub it with garlic and oil and place it in a pan suitable for your air fryer. Add the onion slices, sundried tomatoes, fennel, olives, rosemary and sprinkle with chili flakes; transfer to the air fryer and cook at 380°F for 10 minutes. Divide the fish and vegetables among plates and serve.

178. Hawaiian Salmon

INGREDIENTS | Servings: 2

- ½ tsp. ginger, grated
- 20 ounces canned pineapple pieces and juice
- 2 tsp. garlic powder
- 1 tbsp. balsamic vinegar
- salt and black pepper to taste
- 1 tsp. onion powder
- 2 medium salmon fillets, boneless

DIRECTIONS | Ready in about: 20 min

Season salmon with garlic powder, onion powder, salt and black pepper, rub well, transfer to a heatproof dish that fits your air fryer, add ginger and minced and mix gently. Pour the vinegar all over, put in the air fryer and cook at 350°F for 10 minutes. Divide everything between plates and serve.

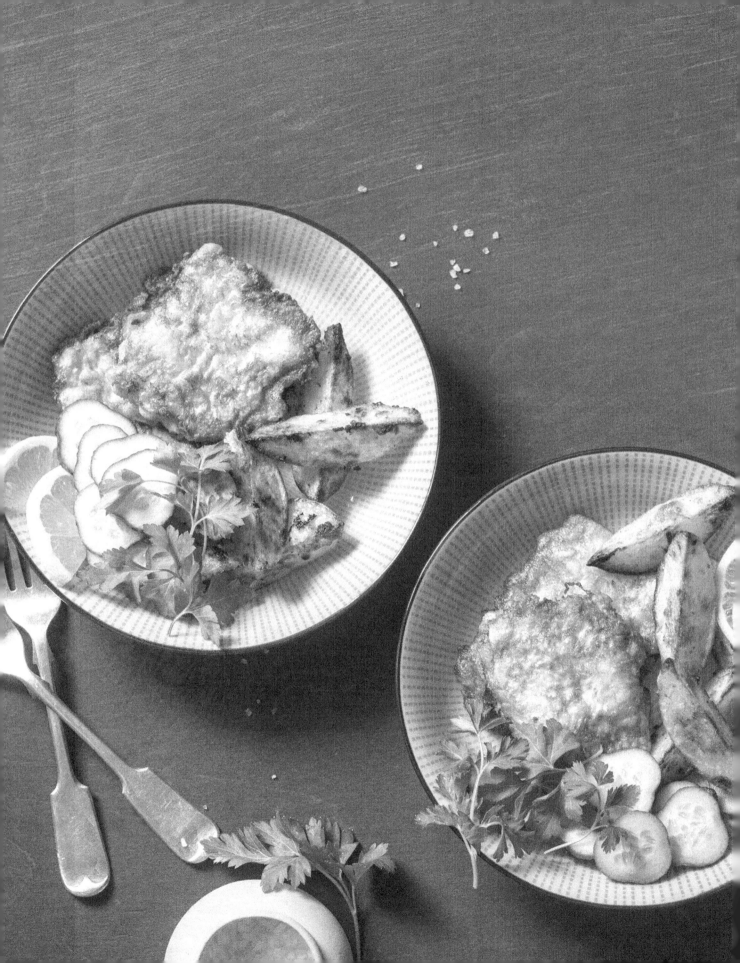

179. Honey Sea Bass

INGREDIENTS | **Servings:** 2

- zest from ½ orange, grated
- 2 sea bass fillets
- juice from ½ orange
- 2 tbsp. mustard
- 1 pinch of salt and black pepper
- 2 tsp. honey
- ½ pound canned lentils, drained
- 2 tbsp. olive oil
- 1 small bunch of dill, chopped
- 1 small bunch of parsley, chopped
- 2 ounces watercress

DIRECTIONS | **Ready in about:** 20 min

Spice the fish fillets with salt and pepper, add the zest and orange juice, rub with 1 tbsp. oil, honey and mustard, rubbing, transfer into an air fryer to air and bake at 350°F for 10 minutes, turning on the medium. Meanwhile, put the lentils in a saucepan, heat them over medium heat, add the rest of the oil, watercress, dill and parsley, mix well and divide into plates. Add the fish fillets and serve immediately.

180. Juicy Salmon and Asparagus Parcels

INGREDIENTS | **Servings:** 2

- 4 asparagus stalks
- 2 salmon fillets
- ¼ cup champagne
- ¼ cup white sauce
- salt and black pepper, to taste
- 1 tsp. olive oil

DIRECTIONS | **Ready in about:** 18 min

Preheat the air fryer to 355°F and grease an air fryer basket. Mix all the ingredients together in a portable bowl and divide the mixture evenly over 2 foil papers. Place the foil in the air fryer basket and cook for about 13 minutes. Serve on a plate and serve hot.

181. Lemon Garlic Shrimp

INGREDIENTS | **Servings:** 2

- 8 ounces medium shelled and deveined shrimp
- 1 medium lemon
- 2 tbsp. unsalted butter, melted
- ½ tsp. minced garlic
- ½ tsp. Old Bay seasoning
- 1 zest lemon and then cut in half

DIRECTIONS | **Ready in about:** 12 min

Spot the shrimp in an enormous bowl and squeeze the juice of ½ lemon over it. Add lemon zest in the bowl with the rest of the ingredients. Stir the shrimp until they are completely covered. Pour it into the 6 "round baking sheet. Insert it into the air fryer basket. Set the temperature to 400°F and set the timer for 6 minutes. The shrimp will be bright pink when fully cooked. Serve hot with a sauce in the pan.

182. Mackerel with Sweet Potatoes

INGREDIENTS | **Servings:** 2

- 2 tbsp. butter
- 1 onion
- 2 sweet potatoes
- 2 cups corn
- 1 lb. mackerel fish
- 2 cups chicken broth
- salt and pepper to taste
- 1 tbsp. cornstarch
- ½ tsp. red pepper flakes

DIRECTIONS | **Ready in about:** 16 min

Add butter and onion into the air fryer pot. Add the chicken broth and mix well. Combine the sweet potatoes, corn, salt and pepper, mackerel fish, cornstarch and red pepper flakes. Bake at 300°F for 20 minutes. Serve and enjoy.

183. Mushrooms with Shrimps

INGREDIENTS | **Servings:** 2

- 1 tbsp. olive oil
- 2 tbsp. chili powder
- 2 tbsp. cardamom seeds
- 2 cups mushrooms
- 1 lb. shrimps
- 1 onion, chopped
- 2 limes
- 2 tbsp. fish sauce
- 2 tomatoes

DIRECTIONS | **Ready in about:** 20 min

Add oil and tomatoes into the air fryer pot. Combine the vegetable broth, lime, onion, mushrooms, cardamom seeds and chili powder. Add the shrimp. Bake at 300°F for 15 minutes. When it's ready, help yourself and enjoy!

184. Quick and Easy Shrimp

INGREDIENTS | **Servings:** 2
- 1 tbsp. olive oil
- ½ pound tiger shrimp
- ½ tsp. old bay seasoning
- salt, to taste
- ¼ tsp. cayenne pepper
- ¼ tsp. smoked paprika

DIRECTIONS | **Ready in about:** 25 min

Set the air-fryer temperature to 390°F and grease a fryer basket. Combine all ingredients in an enormous bowl until well combined. Spot the shrimp in the air fryer basket and cook for about 5 minutes. Serve and serve hot.

185. Salmon and Lemon Relish

INGREDIENTS | **Servings:** 2
- salt and black pepper to taste
- 1 tbsp. olive oil
- 2 salmon fillets, boneless

For the relish:
- 1 shallot, chopped
- 1 tbsp. lemon juice
- 1 Meyer lemon, cut in wedges and then sliced
- ¼ cup olive oil
- 2 tbsp. parsley, chopped

DIRECTIONS | **Ready in about:** 40 min

Spice the salmon with salt and pepper, rub it with 1 tbsp. of oil, put it in the basket of the air fryer and cook at 320°F for 20 minutes, turning the fish in half. Meanwhile, in a bowl, combine the shallot with the lemon juice, a pinch of salt and black pepper, mix and let stand 10 minutes. In another bowl, combine the marinated shallot with the lemon wedges, salt, pepper, parsley and ¼ cup of oil and mix well. Divide the salmon between plates, garnish with the lemon sauce and serve.

186. Salmon and Orange Marmalade

INGREDIENTS | **Servings:** 2
- 2 lemons, sliced
- 1-pound wild salmon, skinless, boneless and cubed
- 1 pinch of salt and black pepper
- ¼ cup balsamic vinegar
- ⅓ cup orange marmalade
- ¼ cup of orange juice

DIRECTIONS | **Ready in about:** 25 min

Heat a pot of vinegar over medium heat, add the marmalade and orange juice, mix, bring to a boil, cook for 1 minute and remove from the heat. Place the diced salmon and lemon slices on the skewers, season with salt and black pepper, spread with half of the orange marmalade mixture, place in the air fryer basket and cook at 360°F for 3 minutes on each side. Brush the skewers with the remaining vinegar, divide among plates and serve immediately with a salad garnish.

187. Salmon Patties

INGREDIENTS | **Servings:** 2
- 2 (5 ounces) pouches cooked pink salmon
- 1 large egg
- ¼ cup ground pork rinds
- 2 tbsp. full-fat mayonnaise
- 2 tsp. chili sauce
- 1 tsp. chili powder

DIRECTIONS | **Ready in about:** 18 min

Mix all the ingredients in an enormous bowl and form four meatballs. Spot the meatballs in the air fryer basket. Set the air-fryer temperature to 400°F and set the timer for 8 minutes. Carefully turn each cake halfway through the cooking time. When fully cooked, the meatball will be crispy on the outside.

188. Sweet Cashew Sticks

INGREDIENTS | **Servings:** 2
- 1 tbsp. coconut oil, melted
- 2 (6 ounces) tuna steaks
- ½ tsp. garlic powder
- 2 tsp. black sesame seeds
- 2 tsp. white sesame seeds

DIRECTIONS | **Ready in about:** 12 min

Brush each tuna steak with coconut oil and sprinkle with powdered garlic. In a large bowl, toss the sesame seeds together, then shred each tuna steak, covering the steak as completely as possible. Place the tuna steaks in the basket of the air fryer. Set the air-fryer temperature to 400°F and set the timer for 8 minutes. Flip the steaks partially through the cooking time. The steaks will be cooked to an internal temperature of 145°F. Serve hot.

189. Shrimp and Cauliflower

INGREDIENTS | **Servings:** 2

- 1 tbsp. butter
- 1 cauliflower head, riced
- ¼ cup heavy cream
- cooking spray
- 1 pound shrimp, peeled and deveined
- 8 ounces mushrooms, roughly chopped
- salt and black pepper to the taste
- 1 pinch of red pepper flakes
- 2 garlic cloves, minced
- 1 tbsp. chives, chopped
- ½ cup beef stock
- 4 bacon slices, cooked and crumbled
- 1 tbsp. parsley, finely chopped

DIRECTIONS | **Ready in about:** 22 min

Spice the shrimp with salt and pepper, drizzle with cooking oil, put in the air fryer and cook at 360°F for 7 minutes. Meanwhile, heat a pan with the butter over medium heat, add the mushrooms, mix and cook for 3-4 minutes. Add the garlic, the cauliflower rice, the pepper flakes, the broth, the cream, the chives, the parsley, the salt and the pepper, mix, cook a few minutes and remove from the heat. Divide the shrimp among plates, add the cauliflower mixture on the side, sprinkle with bacon and serve.

190. Simple Buttery Cod

INGREDIENTS | **Servings:** 2

- 2 tbsp. salted butter, melted
- ½ medium lemon, sliced
- 2 (4 ounces) cod fillets
- 1 tsp. Old Bay seasoning

DIRECTIONS | **Ready in about:** 12 min

Place the cod fillets in an 18 cm round baking dish. Brush each drizzle with butter and sprinkle with Old Bay Seasoning. Place two lemon slices on each fillet. Use foil to cover the baking sheet and place it in the air fryer basket. Set the air-fryer temperature to 350°F and set the timer for 8 minutes. Turn halfway through the cooking time. When it's cooked, the internal temperature of at least 145°F. Serve hot.

191. Snapper Fillets and Veggies

INGREDIENTS | **Servings:** 2

- 1 tbsp. olive oil
- 2 red snapper fillets, boneless
- ½ cup red bell pepper, chopped
- ½ cup leeks, chopped
- ½ cup green bell pepper, chopped
- salt and black pepper to taste
- 1 splash of white wine
- 1 tsp. tarragon, dried

DIRECTIONS | **Ready in about:** 24 min

In a heat-resistant dish suitable for your air fryer, mix the fish fillets with salt, pepper, oil, green pepper, red pepper, leek, tarragon and wine, well toss, place in a preheated 350°F air fryer and cook for 14 minutes, turning the fish fillets in halfway. Divide the fish and vegetables between plates and serve hot.

192. Squid and Guacamole

INGREDIENTS | **Servings:** 2

- 1 tbsp. olive oil
- salt and black pepper to taste
- 2 medium squids, tentacles separated and tubes scored lengthwise
- juice from 1 lime
- For the guacamole:
- 1 tbsp. coriander, chopped
- 2 avocados, pitted, peeled and chopped
- 2 red chilies, chopped
- juice from 2 limes
- 1 red onion, chopped
- 1 tomato, chopped

DIRECTIONS | **Ready in about:** 16 min

Season squid and squid tentacles with salt, pepper and olive oil all over, put in your air fryer basket and bake at 360°F for 3 minutes on each side. Transfer the squid to a bowl, drizzle with lemon juice and mix. Meanwhile, put the avocado in a bowl, mash it with a fork, add the cilantro, peppers, tomato, onion and 2 lime juice and mix. Divide the calamari between plates, garnish with guacamole and serve.

193. Steamed Salmon with Dill Sauce

INGREDIENTS | **Servings:** 2
- 2 (6 ounces) salmon fillets
- 1 cup water
- ½ cup Greek yogurt
- 2 tsp. olive oil
- ½ cup sour cream
- 2 tbsp. fresh dill, chopped and divided
- salt to taste

DIRECTIONS | **Ready in about:** 27 min

Preheat the air fryer to 285°F and grease a fryer basket. Place the water at the bottom of the air tank. Sprinkle the salmon with olive oil and season with a pinch of salt. Spot the salmon in the air fryer and cook for about 11 minutes. Meanwhile, combine the rest of the ingredients in a bowl to make the dill sauce. Serve the salmon with a dill sauce.

194. Stuffed Salmon

INGREDIENTS | **Servings:** 2
- 1 tbsp. olive oil
- 2 salmon fillets, skinless and boneless
- 5 ounces tiger shrimp, peeled, deveined and chopped
- 3 green onions, chopped
- 6 mushrooms, chopped
- 2 cups spinach, torn
- salt and black pepper to taste
- ¼ cup macadamia nuts, toasted and chopped

DIRECTIONS | **Ready in about:** 30 min

Warm a pan with half the oil over medium-high heat, add the mushrooms, onion, salt and pepper, stir and cook for 4 minutes. Add the macadamia nuts, spinach and shrimp, mix, cook for 3 minutes and remove from heat. Make a longitudinal incision in each salmon fillet, season with salt and pepper, divide the mixed spinach and shrimp into incisions and rub with the rest of the olive oil. Spot it in your air fryer basket and cook at 360°F and cook for 10 minutes, turning halfway. Divide the stuffed salmon between the plates and serve.

195. Super-Simple Scallops

INGREDIENTS | **Servings:** 2
- 1 tbsp. butter, melted
- salt and black pepper, to taste
- ¾ pound sea scallops
- ½ tbsp. fresh thyme, minced

DIRECTIONS | **Ready in about:** 15 min

Set the air-fryer temperature to 390°F and grease a fryer basket. Combine all ingredient together in a portable bowl and toss well to coat. Spot the scallops in the air fryer basket and cook for about 4 minutes. Serve hot.

196. Swordfish and Mango Salsa

INGREDIENTS | **Servings:** 2
- salt and black pepper to the taste
- 2 medium swordfish steaks
- 2 tsp. avocado oil
- 1 mango, chopped
- 1 tbsp. cilantro, chopped
- 1 pinch of onion powder
- 1 pinch of cumin
- 1 pinch of garlic powder
- ½ tbsp. balsamic vinegar
- 1 orange, peeled and sliced
- 1 avocado, pitted, peeled and chopped

DIRECTIONS | **Ready in about:** 16 min

Spice the fish fillets with salt, pepper, garlic powder, onion powder and cumin and rub with half of the oil, place in the air fryer and cook at 360°F for 6 minutes turning half. Meanwhile, in a bowl, mix avocado with mango, coriander, balsamic vinegar, salt, pepper and remaining oil and mix well. Fish Divide among plates, sauce garnish with mango and serve with the slice of orange on the side.

197. Tuna Fish with Squash

INGREDIENTS | **Servings:** 2

- 1 can tuna fish
- 2 cups squash, chopped
- salt to taste
- 2 tbsp. tomato sauce
- 2 cups beans
- 1 tbsp. cumin powder

DIRECTIONS | **Ready in about:** 16 min

Add tuna into the air fryer pot. Combine the pumpkin, tomato sauce, beans and cumin powder. Add the salt. Cook at 300°F for 10 minutes. When it's ready, help yourself and enjoy!

198. Tuna Fish with Tomato Paste

INGREDIENTS | **Servings:** 2

- 4 potatoes
- 4 tomatoes
- ½ cup water
- 1 can tomato paste
- 1 can tuna fish
- salt and pepper to taste
- ½ chopped basil
- 1 tbsp. oil

DIRECTIONS | **Ready in about:** 15 min

Add oil into the air fryer pot. Combine the water, tomato paste, tuna, basil and salt and pepper. Mix well. Add the potatoes and tomatoes. Cook at 300°F for 15 minutes. Serve and enjoy!

199. Tuna Puff Pastry

INGREDIENTS | **Servings:** 2

- 1 egg (white and yolk separated)
- 2 square puff pastry dough, bought ready
- ½ cup tuna tea
- ½ cup chopped tea olives
- ½ cup chopped parsley tea
- salt and pepper to taste

DIRECTIONS | **Ready in about:** 16 min

Preheat the air fryer. Set the timer to 5 minutes and the temperature to 400°F. Mix the tuna with the olives and parsley. Season to taste and set aside. Place half of the filling in each dough and fold it in half. Brush with egg white and close gently. After closing, make two small notches in the upper part of the air outlet. Brush with the egg yolk. Place in the air fryer basket. Set the time to 10 minutes and press the power button.

200. Zucchini with Salmon Fillets

INGREDIENTS | **Servings:** 2

- 2 tbsp. canola oil
- 1 onion, chopped
- 1 zucchini, chopped
- 1 lb. salmon fillets
- 3 cups black beans
- 2 tomatoes, diced
- salt and pepper to taste
- ½ cup corn
- parsley to garnish

DIRECTIONS | **Ready in about:** 14 min

Add oil into the air fryer pot. Combine the salmon fillets, onion, black beans, tomatoes, corn, zucchini and salt and pepper. Cook at 300°F for 10 minutes. When cooked, garnish with parsley and serve.

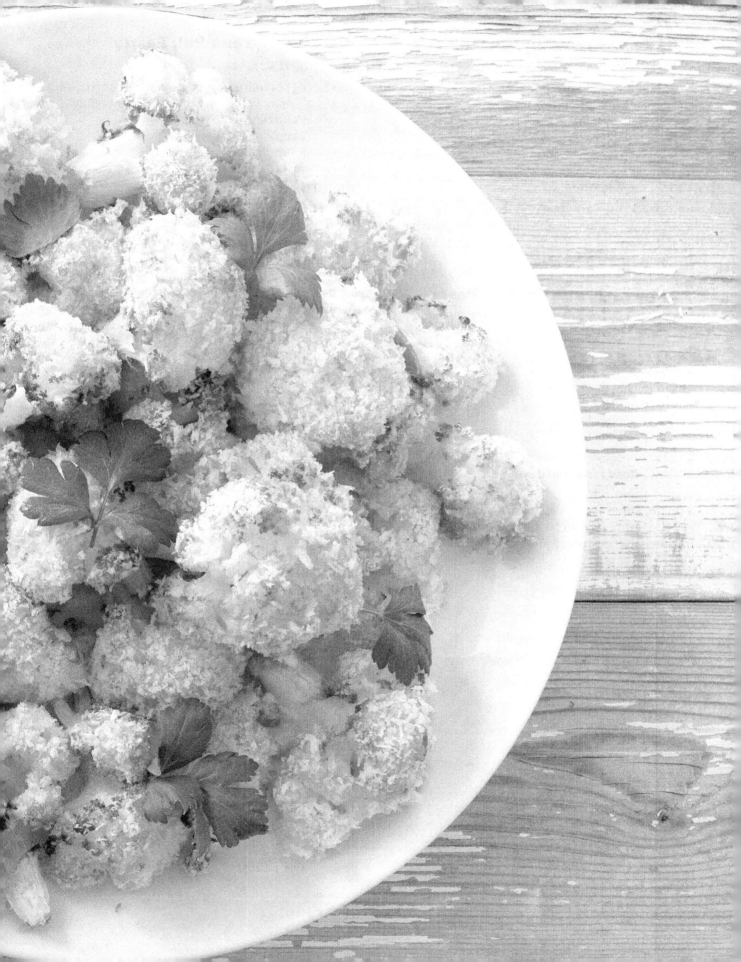

PLANT BASED

201. Beans Burrito

INGREDIENTS | **Servings:** 2
- cooking spray
- 2 cups baked black beans
- ½ red bell pepper, sliced
- 2 tbsp. vegan salsa
- 1 small avocado, peeled, pitted and sliced
- salt and black pepper to taste
- 1/8 cup cashew cheese, grated
- vegan tortillas for serving

DIRECTIONS | **Ready in about:** 20 min

Lubricate your air fryer with cooking spray, add the beans, bell pepper, salsa, salt and pepper, cover and cook at 400°F for 6 minutes. Arrange the tortillas on a work surface, distribute the bean mixture over each, also add the avocado and cashews, roll the burritos, place them in the air fryer, cover and cook at 300°F for another 3 minutes. Divide the burritos between plates and serve.

202. Bell Pepper Oatmeal

INGREDIENTS | **Servings:** 2
- 2 tbsp. canned kidney beans, drained
- 1 cup steel cut oats
- 2 red bell peppers, chopped
- ¼ tsp. cumin, ground
- 1 pinch of sweet paprika
- 4 tbsp. coconut cream
- salt and black pepper to taste

DIRECTIONS | **Ready in about:** 25 min

Heat your air fryer to 360°F, add the oatmeal, beans, peppers, coconut cream, paprika, salt, pepper and cumin, mix, cover and cook for 16 minutes. Divide into bowls and serve.

203. Black Beans Mix Soup

INGREDIENTS | **Servings:** 2
- 4 cups black beans
- 2 zucchinis, chopped
- 3 onions, chopped
- 2 tbsp. olive oil
- salt to taste
- 1 tbsp. oregano
- 1 tbsp. chili powder
- ½ cup green chilies
- cilantro leaves to garnish
- garnish

DIRECTIONS | **Ready in about:** 16 min

Add oil into the air fryer pot. Toss black beans, zucchini, onions, salt, oregano, chili powder, green chilies with salt. Cook at 300°F for 20 minutes. When finished, garnish with cilantro to serve!

204. Black Eyed Peas

INGREDIENTS | **Servings:** 2
- 2 sweet potatoes, sliced
- 1 tbsp. coriander seeds
- 1 tbsp. cumin seeds
- 4 cups black eyed peas
- salt to taste
- 2 garlic cloves
- 2 cups tomato paste
- 1 onion, chopped

DIRECTIONS | **Ready in about:** 14 min

Add tomato paste into the air fryer pot. Mix the onion, garlic, salt, black peas, seeds cumin and coriander seeds. Add the sweet potatoes. Cook at 300°F for 10 minutes. When it's ready, serve!

205. Broccoli and Mushrooms Mix

INGREDIENTS | **Servings:** 2
- 1 broccoli head, florets separated
- 10 ounces mushrooms, halved
- 1 garlic clove, minced
- 1 yellow onion, chopped
- 1 tbsp. balsamic vinegar
- 1 tbsp. olive oil
- 1 pinch of red pepper flakes
- 1 tsp. basil, dried
- salt and black pepper
- 1 avocado, peeled, pitted and roughly cubed

DIRECTIONS | **Ready in about:** 38 min

In a portable bowl, combine the mushrooms with the broccoli, onion, garlic and avocado. In another bowl, combine the vinegar, oil, salt, pepper and basil and mix well. Pour over the vegetables, toss to coat, set aside for 30 minutes, transfer to the air fryer basket and cook at 350°F for 8 minutes, divide between plates and serve with chili flakes.

206. Broccoli Mix

INGREDIENTS | **Servings:** 2
- 2 cups vegetable broth
- 3 cups broccoli
- 1 tbsp. cumin powder
- 1 tbsp. cayenne powder
- 3 green onion
- salt to taste

DIRECTIONS | **Ready in about:** 12 min

Add vegetable broth into the air fryer pot. Combine broccoli, cumin powder, cayenne pepper powder, green onion and salt. Bake at 300°F for 20 minutes. When it's ready, serve and enjoy!

207. Brussels Sprouts and Tomatoes

INGREDIENTS | **Servings:** 2
- salt and black pepper to taste
- 1 pound Brussels sprouts, trimmed
- 6 cherry tomatoes, halved
- 1 tbsp. olive oil
- ¼ cup green onions, chopped

DIRECTIONS | **Ready in about:** 15 min

Spice the Brussels sprouts with salt and pepper, put them in the air fryer and bake at 350°F for 10 minutes. Transfer them to a bowl, add salt, pepper, cherry tomatoes, the onions greens and olive oil, mix well and serve.

208. Chia Pudding

INGREDIENTS | **Servings:** 2
- 2 cups coconut milk
- 1 cup chia seeds
- 2 tbsp. coconut, shredded and unsweetened
- ½ tsp. cinnamon powder
- ½ tsp. vanilla extract
- ¼ cup maple syrup
- 2 tsp. cocoa powder

DIRECTIONS | **Ready in about:** 25 min

In your air fryer, whisk together chia seeds, coconut milk, coconut, maple syrup, cinnamon, cocoa powder and vanilla, stir, cover and cook at 365°F for 15 minutes. Divide the chia pudding between bowls and serve.

209. Chicken and Mushrooms

INGREDIENTS | **Servings:** 2
- ¼ cup oil
- 1 bell pepper, chopped
- 1 onion, chopped
- 2 cups chicken, chopped, breast
- 2 tomatoes, diced
- 3 garlic cloves
- salt and pepper to taste
- 3 drops hot sauce
- 4½ ounce mushrooms

DIRECTIONS | **Ready in about:** 15 min

Add oil into the air fryer pot. Toss the bell pepper, onion, chicken, mushrooms, tomatoes, garlic cloves with salt and pepper. Cook at 300°F for 15 minutes. When done, add the hot sauce and serve!

210. Chicken Tomato Sauce

INGREDIENTS | **Servings:** 2
- 2 cups chicken broth
- 1 lb. chicken breast, chopped
- 2 cups squash, chopped
- salt to taste
- 2 tbsp. tomato sauce
- 2 cups beans
- 1 tbsp. cumin powder

DIRECTIONS | **Ready in about:** 16 min

Add chicken broth into the air fryer pot. Combine the chicken, pumpkin, salt, tomato sauce, beans and cumin seeds. Bake at 300°F for 14 minutes. When it's ready, serve!

211. Crispy French Fries

INGREDIENTS | **Servings:** 2
- 2 tsp olive oil
- 2 medium sweet potatoes
- ½ tsp salt
- black pepper to taste
- ¼ tsp paprika
- ½ tsp garlic powder

DIRECTIONS | **Ready in about:** 15 min

Set air-fryer temperature to 400°F. Sprig the air fryer basket with a little oil. Cut the sweet potatoes into shavings about 1 cm wide. Add the oil, salt, garlic powder, pepper and paprika. Cook for 8 minutes, without overloading the basket. Repeat 2 or 3 times as needed.

212. Frying Potatoes with Butter

INGREDIENTS | **Servings:** 2
- 2 tsp. butter
- fresh parsley
- 2 Russet potatoes
- cooking spray

DIRECTIONS | **Ready in about:** 15 min

Spray the basket with a little oil. Open the potatoes. Make holes with a fork. Add the butter and parsley. Transfer to the basket. Preheat your air fryer until it reaches a temperature of 390°F. Bake for 30 to 40 minutes. Try for about 30 minutes. Enjoy your meal!

213. Homemade French Fries

INGREDIENTS | **Servings:** 2
- 1 tbsp. olive oil
- 1 tsp. salt to season or paprika
- 2½ lb. sliced and sliced potato chips
- salt and pepper to taste

DIRECTIONS | **Ready in about:** 15 min

Put the fries in a bowl with very cold water. Let it soak for at least 30 minutes. Drain completely. Add the oil. Shake them and put them in the air fryer pan. Cook for 15 to 25 minutes. Set to 380°F. Set the time to your preference or the power of your air fryer to 23 minutes.

214. Hot Cabbage Mix

INGREDIENTS | **Servings:** 2
- 1 yellow onion, chopped
- ½ cabbage head, chopped
- salt and black pepper to taste
- 1 dash of Tabasco sauce
- 1 cup coconut cream

DIRECTIONS | **Ready in about:** 30 min

Place the cabbage in a pan suitable for your air fryer. Add onion, salt, pepper, Tabasco sauce and coconut cream, mix, put in the air fryer and cook at 400°F for 20 minutes. Divide between plates and serve.

215. Mediterranean Chickpeas

INGREDIENTS | **Servings:** 2
- 3 shallots, chopped
- cooking spray
- 2 garlic cloves, minced
- ½ tsp. smoked paprika
- ½ tsp. sweet paprika
- 1 tbsp. parsley, chopped
- ½ tsp. cinnamon powder
- 2 tomatoes, chopped
- salt and black pepper to taste
- 2 cup chickpeas, cooked

DIRECTIONS | **Ready in about:** 22 min

Sprig the air fryer with cooking spray and preheat to 365°F. Add the chives, garlic, sweet and smoked paprika, cinnamon, salt, pepper, tomatoes, parsley and chickpeas, mix, cover and cook for 12 minutes. Divide into bowls and serve.

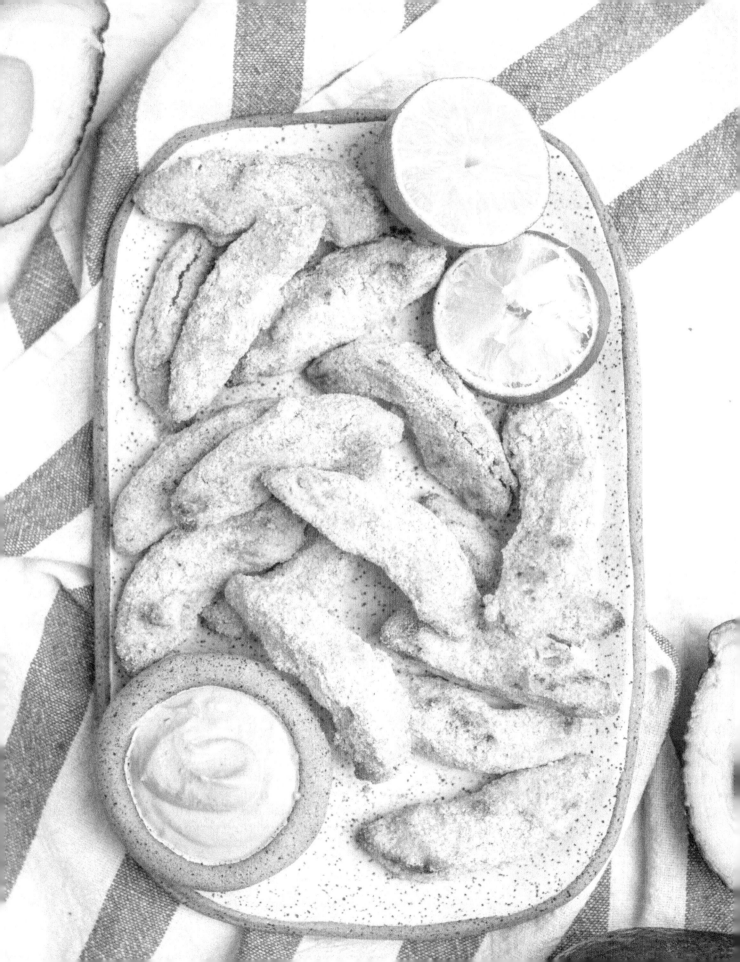

216. Portobello Mini Pizzas

INGREDIENTS | **Servings:** 2

- 2 leaves fresh basil; chopped
- 2 large portobello mushrooms
- ⅔ cup shredded mozzarella cheese
- 1 tbsp. balsamic vinegar
- ½ tsp. garlic powder
- 4 grape tomatoes, sliced
- 2 tbsp. unsalted butter; melted

DIRECTIONS | **Ready in about:** 20 min

Pick up the inside of the mushrooms, leaving only the lids. Butter each lid and sprinkle with garlic powder. Fill each lid with mozzarella and tomato slices. Place each mini pizza in a 6 inch round pan. Place the pan in the air fryer basket. Set the temperature to 380°F and set the timer for 10 minutes. Gently remove the pizzas from the air fryer basket and garnish with the basil and a drizzle of vinegar.

217. Roasted Broccoli Salad

INGREDIENTS | **Servings:** 2

- ½ medium lemon
- 2 tbsp. salted butter; melted.
- 3 cups fresh broccoli florets.
- ¼ cup sliced almonds

DIRECTIONS | **Ready in about:** 15 min

Place broccoli in a 6-inch round baking dish. Pour the butter over the broccoli. Add the almonds and mix. Place the dish in the air fryer basket. Set the temperature to 380°F and set the timer for 7 minutes. Stir halfway through cooking. When the timer rings, grate the lemon over the broccoli and squeeze the juice into the pan. Toss and Serve hot.

218. Spinach Cheese Pie

INGREDIENTS | **Servings:** 2

- ¼ cup heavy whipping cream.
- 1 cup frozen chopped spinach, drained
- 1 cup shredded sharp cheddar cheese.
- 6 large eggs.
- ¼ cup diced yellow onion

DIRECTIONS | **Ready in about:** 30 min

Take a portable bowl, beat the eggs and add the cream. Add the rest of the ingredients to the bowl. Pour into a 6-inch round baking dish. Place in the fryer basket. Set the temperature to 320°F and set the timer for 20 minutes. The eggs will be hard-boiled and lightly browned when cooked. Serve immediately.

219. Sweet Potatoes and Corn

INGREDIENTS | **Servings:** 2

- 2 tbsp. butter
- 1 onion
- 2 sweet potatoes
- 2 cups corn
- 2 cups chicken broth
- salt and pepper to taste
- 1 tbsp. cornstarch
- ½ tsp. red pepper flakes

DIRECTIONS | **Ready in about:** 16 min

Add butter into the air fryer pot. Combine onion, sweet potato, corn, chicken broth, cornstarch, pepper flakes with salt and pepper. Cook at 300°F for 20 minutes. When it's ready, serve!

220. Tomato Frittata

INGREDIENTS | **Servings:** 2

- ½ cup cashew cheese, shredded
- 2 tbsp. flax meal mixed with 3 tbsp. water
- 2 tbsp. yellow onion, chopped
- ¼ cup tomatoes, chopped
- ¼ cup coconut milk
- salt and black pepper to taste

DIRECTIONS | **Ready in about:** 40 min

In a bowl, mix the flax flour with the milk, cheese, salt, pepper, onion and tomatoes, mix well, pour into the pan of your air fryer, cover and cook at 340°F for 30 minutes. Divide the omelet between plates and serve for breakfast.

221. Tomatoes and Basil Mix

INGREDIENTS | **Servings:** 2

- 3 garlic cloves, minced
- 1 bunch basil, chopped
- 1 drizzle of olive oil
- 2 cups cherry tomatoes, halved
- salt and black pepper to taste

DIRECTIONS | **Ready in about:** 24 min

In a pan suitable for your air fryer, combine the tomatoes with the garlic, salt, pepper, basil and oil, mix, place in your air fryer and cook at 320°F for 12 minutes. Divide between plates and serve.

222. Tomatoes Salad

INGREDIENTS | **Servings:** 2

- 1 green onion, chopped
- cooking spray
- 2 tomatoes, halved
- salt and black pepper to taste
- 1 tsp. basil, chopped
- 1 tsp. parsley, chopped
- 1 tsp. oregano, chopped
- 1 cucumber, chopped
- 1 tsp. rosemary, chopped

DIRECTIONS | **Ready in about:** 30 min

Drizzle the tomato halves with the cooking oil, season with salt and pepper, place in the air fryer basket and bake at 320°F for 20 minutes. Transfer the tomatoes to a bowl, add the parsley, basil, oregano, rosemary, cucumber and onion, toss and serve.

223. Vegan Cheese Sandwich

INGREDIENTS | **Servings:** 2

- 2 slices cashew cheese
- 2 slices of vegan bread
- 2 tsp. cashew butter

DIRECTIONS | **Ready in about:** 18 min

Spread the cashew butter on the slices of bread, add the vegan cheese in one slice, on the other, cut in half diagonally, place in the air fryer, cover and cook at 370°F for 8 minutes, turning the medium sandwiches. Serve immediately.

224. Veggie Broth with Cauliflower

INGREDIENTS | **Servings:** 2

- 2 carrots, sliced
- 2 cups vegetable broth
- salt to taste
- 4 cups cauliflower florets
- 2 tbsp. garlic, minced
- 2 tbsp. thyme, dried
- 4 celery stalks
- 1 tbsp. cornstarch

DIRECTIONS | **Ready in about:** 16 min

Add vegetable broth into the air fryer pot. Mix carrot, cauliflower, garlic, thyme, celery stems, cornstarch and salt. Cook at 300°F for 20 minutes. Serve and enjoy!

225. White Mushrooms Mix

INGREDIENTS | **Servings:** 2

- 7 ounces snow peas
- salt and black pepper to taste
- 8 ounces white mushrooms, halved
- 1 tsp. olive oil
- 2 tbsp. coconut aminos
- 1 yellow onion, cut into rings

DIRECTIONS | **Ready in about:** 25 min

In a portable bowl, peas with mushrooms, onion, coconut aminos, oil, salt and pepper, mix well, transfer to a saucepan suitable for your air fryer, place in the air fryer and cook at 350°F for 15 minutes. Divide between plates and serve.

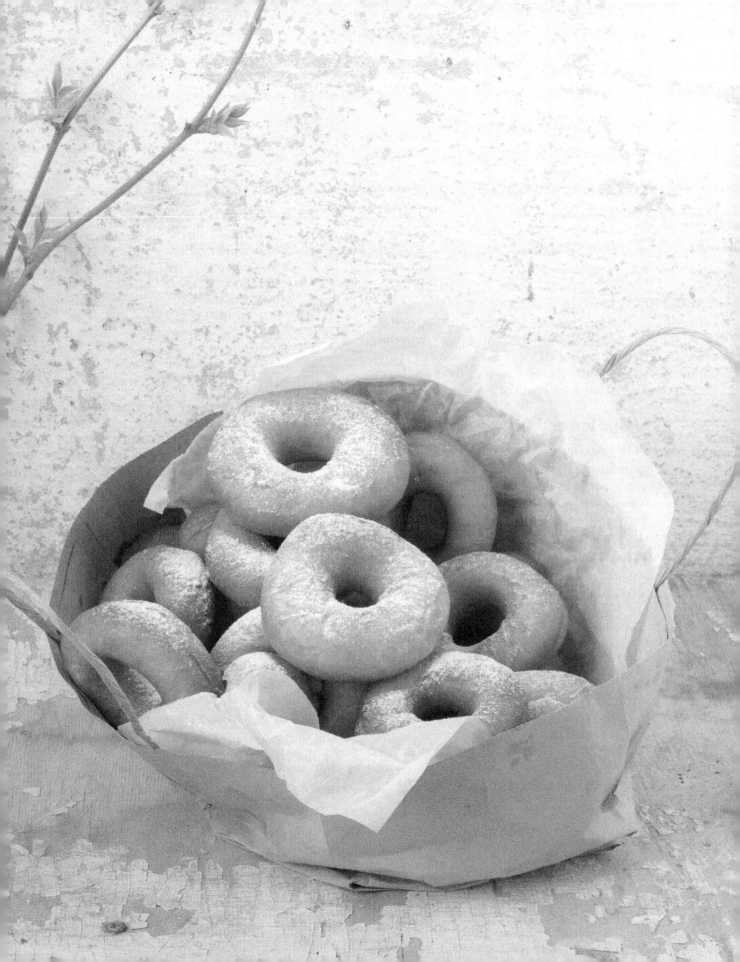

DESSERTS

226. Apple Chips

INGREDIENTS | Servings: 2
- 1 apple
- 1 pinch kosher salt
- ½ tsp. cinnamon
- 1 tbsp. sugar

DIRECTIONS | Ready in about: 1 h 20 min

Heat the air fryer in advance to reach 390°F. Cut the apples lengthwise and place them on a plate with the cinnamon, sugar and salt. Cough. Bake until crisp or about seven to eight minutes. Turn in the middle of the cycle. Transfer to a serving plate and serve.

227. Apples and Wine Sauce

INGREDIENTS | Servings: 2
- 1 tsp. nutmeg, ground
- ½ cup sugar
- 3 apples, cored and cut into wedges
- 1 cup red wine

DIRECTIONS | Ready in about: 30 min

In your air fryer's pan, combine the apples with the nutmeg and other ingredients, mix and cook at 340°F for 20 minutes. Divide into bowls and serve.

228. Apples Mix Dessert

INGREDIENTS | Servings: 2
- 2 cups apples, sliced
- 2 tbsp. lemon juice
- 2 tbsp. sugar
- 2 cups flour
- 2 tbsp. rolled oats
- 2 tbsp. brown sugar
- 2 tbsp. cinnamon powder
- 3 tbsp. butter
- 1 cup nuts, chopped

DIRECTIONS | Ready in about: 19 min

In a portable bowl, include the flour and sugar. Combine the lemon juice, oatmeal, brown sugar, Cinnamon powder, butter and nuts. Pour the batter into the round pan. Bake at 300°F for 15 minutes in the air fryer. When it's ready, place the apples on the cake to serve!

229. Black Cherries Dessert

INGREDIENTS | Servings: 2
- 2 tbsp. butter
- 1 cup milk
- 2 tbsp. sugar
- 2 tbsp. vanilla extract
- 3 eggs
- ¼ tbsp. salt
- 2 cups flour
- 2 cups black cherries
- powdered sugar for dusting

DIRECTIONS | Ready in about: 17 min

Add butter and milk to the bowl. Combine the sugar, vanilla extract, eggs, salt and flour. Spurt the batter into the round baking pan. Bake at 300°F for 15 minutes in the air fryer. When it's ready, top the cake with blueberries and powdered sugar for serving!

230. Brioche Bread

INGREDIENTS | Servings: 2
- 2 tbsp. butter
- 1 loaf brioche bread
- 1 cup pecans (chopped)
- 1 cup half and half
- 1 cup whole milk
- 2 eggs
- 2 cups brown sugar
- 2 tbsp. vanilla extract
- 2 tbsp. cinnamon powder
- 1 pinch salt
- 1 tbsp. nutmeg powder

DIRECTIONS | Ready in about: 22 min

Place the bread in the round baking tray. Add the butter and whole milk to the bowl. Combine half and half, egg, brown sugar, vanilla extract, Cinnamon powder, salt and ground nutmeg. Bake at 300°F for 20 minutes in the air fryer. When it's ready, top the pecans for serving!

231. Cake with Strawberries Cream

INGREDIENTS | Servings: 2
- 16 ounces strawberries (clean and without skin)
- 3 tbsp icing sugar baked at 400°F in the air fryer
- 1 pure butter puff pastry to stretch
- 1 bowl of custard

DIRECTIONS | Ready in about: 25 min

Unroll and put the puff pastry on the baking sheet. Prick the bottom with a fork and spread the cream. Arrange the strawberries in a circle and sprinkle with icing sugar. Bake in an air fryer at 400°F for 15 minutes. Remove the cake from the fryer with the tongs and let cool. Sprinkle with icing sugar when it's done, add a little whipped cream and serve.

232. Chocolate Banana

INGREDIENTS | Servings: 2
- 10 chocolate chips
- 2 bananas

DIRECTIONS | Ready in about: 12 min

Use a knife to cut the banana deeply lengthwise. Be careful, however, not to completely cut the banana. Now fill the chocolate chips in this slot. Place the plantains in the coated pan of your air fryer and bake for 6 minutes at 350°F Cut the banana into small pieces and serve.

233. Chocolate Chips

INGREDIENTS | Servings: 2
- 3 egg yolks
- 2 tbsp. sugar
- 1 cup milk
- 2 cups flour
- 2 cups cheese
- 2 cups grounded coffee
- 2 tbsp. cocoa powder
- 1 cup chocolate chips

DIRECTIONS | Ready in about: 20 min

Add flour and milk to the bowl. Stir in the egg yolks, sugar, cheese, coffee, cocoa powder and chocolate chips. Pour the batter into the round pan. Bake at 300°F for 15 minutes in the air fryer. Serve and enjoy!

234. Chocolate Mixed Cocoa

INGREDIENTS | Servings: 2
- 2 cups chocolate, chopped
- 1½ cup butter
- ½ tsp. salt
- 2 egg yolks
- 1 cup cocoa powder

DIRECTIONS | Ready in about: 17 min

In a portable bowl, include chocolate and butter. Combine the salt, egg yolks and cocoa powder. Pour the batter into the round baking pan. Bake at 300°F for 15 minutes in the air fryer. When it's ready, serve and enjoy!

235. Coconut Mix Dessert

INGREDIENTS | **Servings:** 2

- 2 tbsp. butter
- 2 cups sugar
- 3 eggs
- 2 tbsp. vanilla extract
- 2 tbsp. almond extract
- 2 cups flour
- 2 tbsp. baking powder
- 1 pinch salt
- 2 cups milk
- 2 cups shredded coconut

Frosting:

- 2 cups cream
- 2 tbsp. butter
- 2 tbsp. vanilla extract
- 1 cup sugar

DIRECTIONS | **Ready in about:** 17 min

Include butter and sugar to the bowl. Combine the eggs, vanilla extract, almond extract, flour, baking powder, salt, milk and grated coconut. Pour the batter into the round pan. Bake at 300°F for 15 minutes in the air fryer. Make the icing: mix the cream, butter, vanilla extract and sugar in the bowl. When the cake is done, top it with the frosting to serve!

236. Delicious Buttercream

INGREDIENTS | **Servings:** 2

- 1 cup sugar
- 3 tbsp. almond flour
- 3 egg whites
- 4 tbsp. granulated sugar
- 2 tbsp. food color (any)
- 4 cups buttercream for filling (any)

DIRECTIONS | **Ready in about:** 24 min

In a portable bowl, include the flour and sugar. Combine the egg whites, sugar and food coloring. Pour the batter into the round pan. Bake at 300°F for 20 minutes in the air fryer. When finished, pour over the buttercream to serve!

237. Honey Cake

INGREDIENTS | **Servings:** 2

- 2 cups butter
- 2 cups flour
- 2 tbsp. sugar
- 1 tbsp. brown sugar
- 2 cups honey
- 3 egg whites
- 1 tbsp. baking powder
- 1 cup chopped pistachios
- 1 cup chopped almonds

DIRECTIONS | **Ready in about:** 12 min

Add the butter and flour to the bowl. Combine the sugar, brown sugar, egg whites and yeast. Pour the mixture into the round baking pan. Bake at 300°F for 10 minutes in the air fryer. When it's ready, cover the cake with honey and garnish with pistachios. Add almonds to serve and enjoy!

238. Kiwi and Strawberry Mix

INGREDIENTS | **Servings:** 2

- 2 cups flour
- 2 tbsp. baking powder
- 1 pinch salt
- 2 cups sugar
- 2 tbsp. butter
- 2 tbsp. vanilla extract
- 2 eggs
- 2 kiwi, sliced
- 2 cups strawberries, sliced
- 2 cups whipped cream

DIRECTIONS | **Ready in about:** 17 min

In a portable bowl, include the flour and baking powder. Combine the salt, sugar, butter, vanilla extract and eggs. Pour the batter into the round pan. Bake at 300°F for 15 minutes in the air fryer. When finished, spread the whipped cream on the cake. Serve kiwi and strawberries!

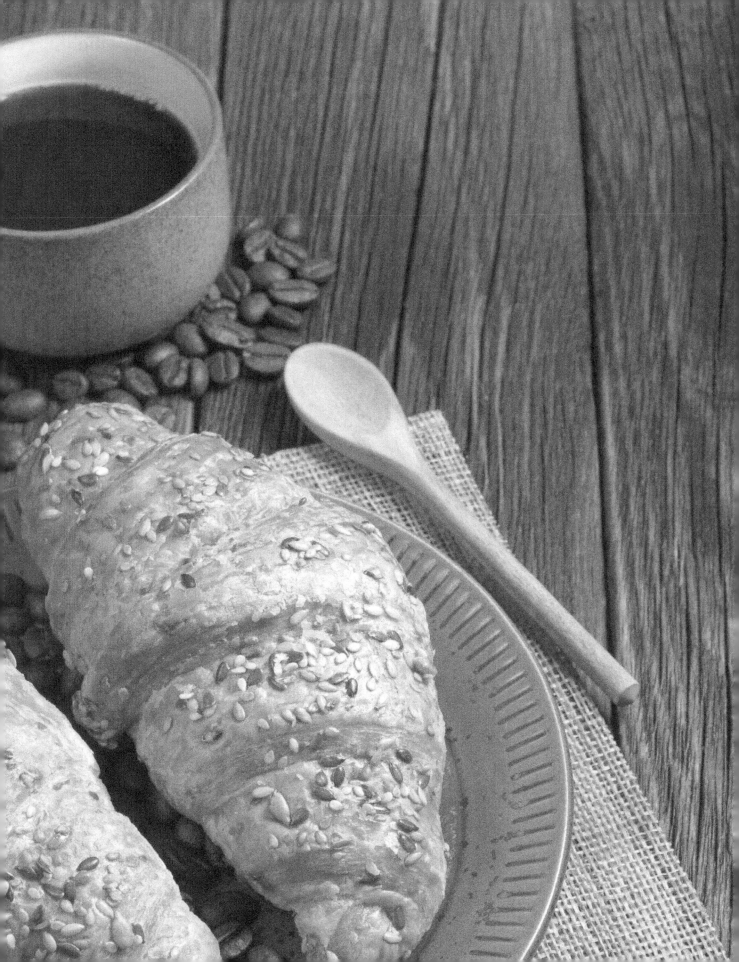

239. Oats and Blueberries Mix

INGREDIENTS | **Servings:** 2
- 2 tbsp. brown sugar
- 1 cup butter
- 1 tbsp. vanilla extract
- 2 eggs
- 2 cups flour
- 1 pinch salt
- 1 tbsp. baking soda
- 3 cups oats
- 1 cup blueberries

DIRECTIONS | **Ready in about:** 17 min

Add the brown sugar and butter to the bowl. Combine the vanilla extract, eggs, flour, salt, baking soda and oatmeal. Add the blueberries. Pour the batter into the round pan. Bake at 300°F for 15 minutes in the air fryer. When it's ready, serve!

240. Pecans Filled Dessert

INGREDIENTS | **Servings:** 2
Pie Crust:
- 2 cups flour
- 1 cup vegetable shortening
- 2 tbsp. butter
- 2 egg
- 2 tbsp. white vinegar

Filling:
- 1 cup sugar
- 1 cup brown sugar
- 2 tbsp. corn syrup
- 2 tbsp. vanilla extract
- 2 tbsp. butter
- 1 cup pecans, chopped

DIRECTIONS | **Ready in about:** 18 min

Add the flour and shortening to the bowl. Mix the butter, eggs and white vinegar. Pour the batter into the round pan. Bake at 300°F for 15 minutes in the air fryer. Prepare the filling: Mix sugar, brown sugar, the vanilla extract, butter and nuts in a bowl. Pour in the garnish to serve when the crust is ready.

241. Raspberry Jam Delight

INGREDIENTS | **Servings:** 2
- 2 cups butter
- 2 tbsp. vanilla extract
- 2 cups flour
- 1 pinch salt
- 1 cup raspberry jam
- 1 cup dried fruit (any)
- 1 cup almonds, sliced
- 1 cup sugar

DIRECTIONS | **Ready in about:** 18 min

Add the butter and flour to the air fryer pot. Combine the vanilla extract, salt, nuts, almonds and sugar. Pour the batter into the round pan. Bake at 300°F for 15 minutes in the air fryer. When it's ready, apply the raspberry jam and garnish the almonds for serving.

242. Red Velvet Cake

INGREDIENTS | **Servings:** 2
- 2 cups flour
- 2 tbsp. sugar
- 1 tbsp. baking soda
- 1 pinch salt
- 2 tbsp. cocoa powder
- 1 tbsp. oil
- 1 cup buttermilk
- 2 eggs
- red food coloring
- 2 tbsp. vanilla extract
- cream cheese for frosting
- 1 cups pecan, chopped

DIRECTIONS | **Ready in about:** 25 min

Include flour and sugar to the bowl. Combine the baking soda, salt, cocoa powder, oil and buttermilk, eggs, red food coloring and vanilla extract. Pour the batter into the round pan. Bake at 300°F for 15 minutes in the air fryer. When it's ready, top it with whipped cream. Garnish the nuts to serve!

243. Saltine Crackers Mix

INGREDIENTS | Servings: 2
- 1 tbsp. oil
- 30 saltine crackers
- 1 cup butter
- 2 tbsp. brown sugar
- 1 cup chocolate chips

DIRECTIONS | Ready in about: 17 min

Add the oil and butter to the bowl. Stir in crackers, brown sugar and chocolate chips. Pour the batter into the round pan. Bake at 300°F for 15 minutes in the air fryer. Serve and enjoy!

244. Simple Cake

INGREDIENTS | Servings: 2
- 1 cup flour (all-purpose)
- 1 tbsp. baking powder
- 1 pinch salt
- 2 cups sugar
- 2 tbsp. butter
- 2 tbsp. vanilla extract
- 1 cup milk

DIRECTIONS | Ready in about: 17 min

Include flour and baking powder to the bowl. Combine salt, sugar, butter, vanilla extract and milk. Make sure there are no lumps in the dough. Pour the batter into the round pan. Bake at 300°F for 15 minutes in the air fryer. When it's ready, serve and enjoy!

245. Simple Sweet Sheets

INGREDIENTS | Servings: 2
- 2 cups butter
- 1 cup sugar
- ½ tsp. salt
- 3 apples, chopped
- ½ cup brandy (any)
- 3 phyllo dough sheets

DIRECTIONS | Ready in about: 18 min

In a portable bowl, include the butter and sugar. Combine the salt, apples and brandy. Place the leaves in the round pan Pour the batter into the tray. Bake at 300°F for 15 minutes in the air fryer. Serve and enjoy!

246. Soft Rice

INGREDIENTS | Servings: 2
- 1 cup white rice
- 1 cup whole milk
- 1 tbsp. lemon juice
- 1 cup white sugar
- 2 egg yolks, beaten
- 2 tbsp. vanilla extract
- 2 tbsp. corn flour

DIRECTIONS | Ready in about: 17 min

Add white rice to the air fryer. Combine the whole milk, lemon juice, white sugar, egg yolks, vanilla extract and cornmeal. Bake at 300°F for 15 minutes. Serve and enjoy!

247. Sweet Potato Dessert

INGREDIENTS | Servings: 2
- 3 sweet potatoes, mashed
- 2 tbsp. sugar
- 2 eggs
- 2 tbsp. vanilla extract
- 2 tbsp. cinnamon powder
- 1 pinch salt
- 2 cups evaporated milk
- 1 pie crust
- 1 cup whipped cream
- 2 tbsp. maple syrup
- 2 tbsp. sugar

DIRECTIONS | Ready in about: 18 min

Add the sugar and eggs to the bowl. Combine the sweet potatoes, vanilla extract, ground cinnamon, salt and evaporated milk. Place the cake batter in the round pan and pour the batter. Bake at 300°F for 15 minutes in the air fryer. Meanwhile, make the filling: mix the whipped cream, maple syrup and sugar. When the cake is done, cover with topping to serve!

248. Vermicelli Mix

INGREDIENTS | **Servings:** 2
- 3 cups vermicelli
- 2 cups milk
- 1 cup sugar
- 1 tbsp. cardamom powder

DIRECTIONS | **Ready in about:** 23 min

Add the milk and the Vermicelli to the frying pan. Combine the sugar and the cardamom powder. Bake at 300°F for 20 minutes. Serve and enjoy!

249. Walnut Milk

INGREDIENTS | **Servings:** 2
- 2 cups walnut powder
- 2 cups milk
- 1 tsp. gelatin
- 2 tbsp. custard powder
- 3 tbsp. powdered sugar
- 3 tbsp. unsalted butter

DIRECTIONS | **Ready in about:** 23 min

Boil the milk and the sugar in a pan and add the custard powder followed by the walnut powder and stir till you get a thick mixture. Add the gelatin and mix the ingredients well. Preheat the air-fryer to 300°F for five minutes. Place the dish in the basket and reduce the temperature to 250°F. Cook for ten minutes and set aside to cool!

250. White Chocolate

INGREDIENTS | **Servings:** 2
- 2 tbsp. butter
- 1 cup sugar
- 2 tbsp. vanilla extract
- 2 cups flour
- 1 pinch salt
- 2 cups white chocolate, melted

DIRECTIONS | **Ready in about:** 18 min

In a portable bowl, include butter and sugar. Combine the sugar, vanilla extract, salt, flour and white chocolate. Spurt the batter into the round baking pan. Bake at 300°F for 15 minutes in the air fryer. When it's ready, serve and enjoy!

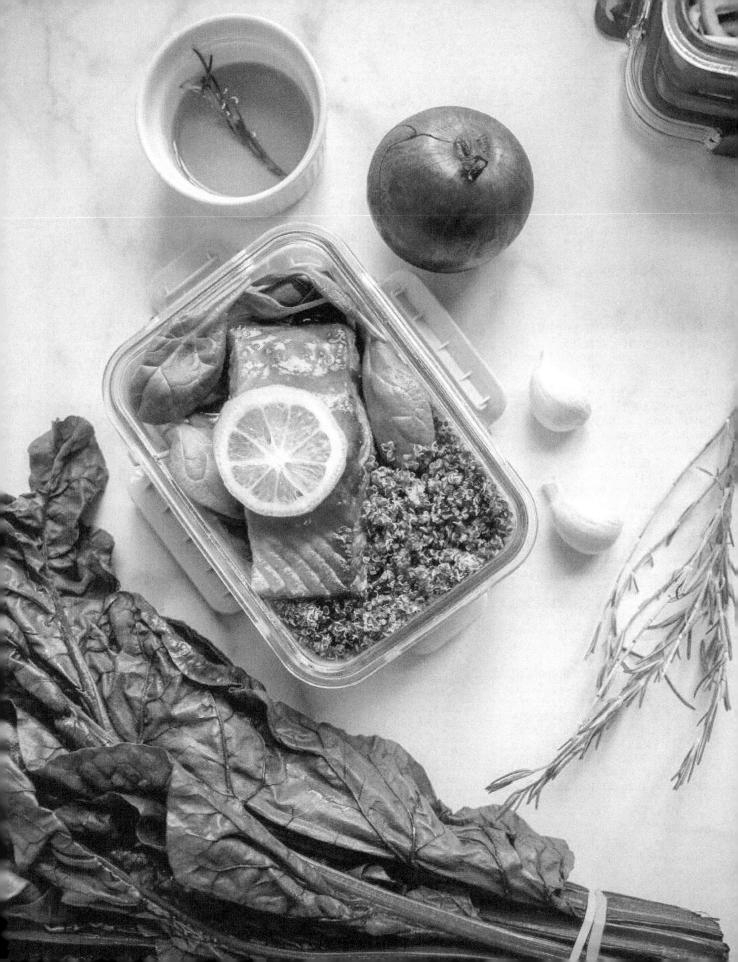

INGREDIENTS INDEX

A

almonds; 42; 65; 154; 157; 217; 235; 237; 241
anise; 144; 148
apples; 133; 226; 227; 228; 245
artichokes; 77
arugula; 84
asparagus; 1; 4; 180
avocado; 1; 7; 46; 49; 50; 73; 95; 113; 125; 151; 192; 196; 201; 205

B

bacon; 5; 37; 38; 60; 73; 74; 75; 98; 189
baking powder; 29; 235; 238; 244
balsamic vinegar; 91; 196
banana; 52; 70; 232
basil; 43; 63; 78; 103; 105; 122; 128; 198; 205; 216; 221; 222
bay leaf; 45; 119; 160
beans; 7; 72; 83; 85; 86; 87; 88; 89; 93; 96; 98; 101; 102; 103; 107; 108; 112; 115; 116; 117; 118; 119; 120; 121; 122; 123; 124; 125; 126; 127; 128; 129; 130; 131; 132; 133; 134; 135; 136; 137; 138; 139; 140; 141; 142; 143; 144; 145; 146; 147; 148; 149; 150; 151;152; 153; 154; 155; 156; 157; 158; 159; 160; 161; 162; 163; 164; 165; 166; 167; 168; 169; 170; 171; 172; 173; 174; 175; 176; 177; 178; 179; 180; 181; 182; 183; 184; 185; 186; 187; 188; 189; 190; 191; 192; 193; 194; 195; 196; 197; 198; 199; 200; 201; 202; 203; 204; 205; 206; 207; 208; 209; 210; 211; 212; 213; 214; 215; 216; 217; 218; 219; 220; 221; 222; 223; 224; 225; 226; 227; 228; 229; 230; 231; 232; 233; 234; 235; 236; 237; 238; 239; 240; 241; 242; 243; 244; 245; 246; 247; 248; 249; 250
beef; 48; 72; 76; 77; 78; 79; 80; 81; 82; 83; 84; 85; 86; 87; 88; 89; 90; 91; 93; 97; 98; 99; 100; 102; 107; 109; 112; 113; 115; 116
beer; 32; 102
beets; 6
bell pepper; 47; 88; 201; 209
black olives; 78; 105
blueberries; 239

bread; 1; 5; 11; 30; 31; 32; 33; 37; 43; 62; 130; 223; 230
breadcrumbs; 117; 138; 174
broccoli; 8; 9; 56; 120; 205; 206; 217
brown sugar; 135; 228; 230; 237; 239; 240; 243
butter; 8; 29; 30; 31; 35; 60; 62; 67; 68; 80; 81; 87; 89; 92; 96; 99; 103; 104; 109; 110; 111; 112; 116; 118; 120; 123; 126; 130; 132; 134; 136; 148; 152; 157; 166; 167; 176; 182; 189; 190; 212; 217; 219; 223; 228; 230; 234; 235; 237; 238; 239; 240; 241; 243; 244; 245; 250

C

cabbage; 81; 101; 145; 214
calamari; 192
canola oil; 109
capers; 61; 100; 123
cardamom; 183; 248
carrot; 9; 10; 33; 71; 79; 90; 101; 119; 136; 171; 224
cashew; 223
cashews; 65; 201
cauliflower; 51; 99; 171; 189; 224
cayenne pepper; 38; 83; 91; 118
celery; 34; 90; 119; 163; 171; 224
cheddar; 9; 32; 48; 67; 93
cheese; 3; 5; 10; 11; 30; 32; 33; 36; 37; 38; 39; 41; 43; 46; 47; 48; 52; 55; 57; 59; 60; 62; 78; 85; 87; 93; 95; 97; 117; 120; 128; 142; 153; 220; 223; 233
cherries; 147
chia seeds; 52; 208
chicken; 8; 10; 42; 53; 117; 118; 119; 120; 121; 122; 123; 124; 125; 126; 127; 128; 129; 130; 131; 132; 133; 134; 135; 136; 137; 138; 139; 140; 141; 142; 145; 146; 151; 153; 154; 155; 156; 182; 209; 210; 219
chickpeas; 54; 164; 165; 215
chili paste; 131
chili powder; 65; 66; 95; 96; 107; 156; 161; 166; 183; 203
chives; 58; 60; 67; 131; 143; 144; 189; 215
chocolate; 232; 233; 234; 243; 250

cilantro; 10; 45; 73; 86; 95; 113; 139; 140; 151; 154; 156; 164; 166; 192; 203
cinnamon; 69; 147; 208; 215; 226; 247
cocoa; 208; 233; 234; 242
coconut; 50; 52; 55; 95; 111; 167; 188; 202; 208; 214; 235
cod; 168; 169; 170; 171; 190
coffee; 233
coriander; 69; 164; 196; 204
corn; 57; 58; 59; 86; 149; 182; 200; 219
cornmeal; 59; 246
cornstarch; 40; 106; 115; 131; 146; 171; 182; 219; 224
crackers; 243
cream; 36; 52; 55; 60; 99; 145; 175; 189; 218; 231; 235; 238; 242; 247
cumin; 54; 66; 69; 96; 126; 140; 147; 155; 164; 169; 196; 197; 202; 204; 206; 210
curry powder; 54; 69; 154; 165

D

dill; 72; 99; 141; 173; 179; 193
duck; 144; 147; 148; 149; 150; 152

E

egg; 1; 4; 5; 7; 9; 29; 31; 32; 34; 35; 37; 41; 44; 46; 47; 49; 50; 51; 55; 58; 59; 66; 67; 94; 109; 119; 128; 129; 174; 199; 218; 230; 233; 234; 235; 236; 237; 238; 239; 240; 242; 246; 247
egg whites; 236; 237

F

fennel; 168; 177
fish fillets; 168; 179; 191; 196
flour; 29; 50; 55; 58; 59; 67; 94; 99; 128; 129; 130; 132; 138; 220; 228; 233; 235; 236; 237; 238; 239; 240; 241; 242; 244; 250

G

garlic; 3; 10; 36; 38; 42; 43; 51; 53; 63; 65; 66; 72; 77; 80; 83; 85; 87; 88; 90; 91; 94; 95; 96; 97; 98; 102; 103; 106; 107; 110; 111; 114; 115; 116; 117; 118; 121; 122; 123; 124; 128; 129; 131; 136; 137; 139; 140; 142; 143; 147; 149; 152; 153; 155; 156; 160; 163; 165; 166; 170; 171; 175; 177; 178; 188; 189; 196; 204; 205; 209; 211; 215; 216; 221; 224
ginger; 51; 53; 69; 76; 79; 102; 106; 115; 124; 131; 133; 143; 144; 147; 164; 170; 178
grapes; 168
Greek yogurt; 41
green onions; 123

H

ham; 1; 5
hazelnut; 65
honey; 53; 65; 70; 91; 106; 115; 127; 131; 146; 147; 150; 159; 179; 237
hot sauce; 3; 88; 102; 117; 132; 209

J

jalapeno; 147; 156; 166
Jicama; 86

L

lemon; 41; 49; 51; 57; 66; 72; 73; 77; 78; 80; 84; 86; 89; 103; 104; 105; 110; 112; 113; 119; 120; 121; 123; 125; 130; 132; 135; 136; 137; 138; 141; 142; 158; 166; 174; 175; 176; 181; 185; 186; 190; 192; 217; 228; 246
lentils; 164; 179
lettuce; 45; 73; 95; 113
Linguine; 87

M

macadamia nuts; 65; 194
mango; 196
maple syrup; 102; 133; 208; 247
mayonnaise; 8; 45; 69; 135; 154
milk; 4; 5; 9; 37; 42; 47; 58; 94; 208; 220; 230; 233; 235; 244; 246; 247; 248
mozzarella; 128; 216
mushrooms; 37; 42; 51; 82; 83; 88; 89; 112; 127; 139; 172; 183; 189; 194; 205; 209; 216
mustard; 32; 74; 84; 102; 108; 150; 165; 179

N

Nutella; 64

nutmeg; 76; 227; 230

O

Oats; 239
olive oil; 6; 82; 113; 121; 148; 153; 173; 192; 193; 194; 207
onion; 8; 30; 33; 34; 39; 42; 45; 47; 53; 66; 72; 76; 81; 82; 83; 88; 91; 94; 95; 97; 98; 99; 101; 105; 108; 109; 115; 119; 122; 124; 125; 129; 136; 137; 143; 146; 147; 151; 155; 156; 160; 163; 172; 177; 178; 182; 183; 192; 194; 196; 200; 204; 205; 206; 209; 214; 219; 220; 222
orange; 179; 186; 196
oregano; 61; 63; 68; 77; 83; 85; 96; 111; 129; 142; 160; 161; 203; 222

P

panko; 49; 128
paprika; 32; 35; 38; 40; 45; 57; 63; 65; 68; 72; 95; 125; 129; 202; 211; 215
parsley; 9; 42; 66; 72; 80; 84; 87; 98; 103; 110; 111; 114; 116; 121; 125; 126; 134; 141; 172; 176; 179; 185; 189; 199; 200; 212; 215; 222
peanut oil; 51
peas; 51; 78; 82; 101; 105; 129; 204
pecans; 230
pesto; 157
pine nuts; 41
pistachios; 237
plantains; 232
plum sauce; 170
pork; 76; 95; 96; 99; 101; 104; 105; 106; 107; 108
potatoes; 30; 55; 60; 63; 66; 89; 90; 140; 182; 198; 204; 211; 212; 247
puff pastry; 66; 231
pumpkin; 17; 18; 20; 24; 25; 27; 28; 29; 30; 31; 32; 33; 34; 35; 36; 37; 38; 39; 40; 41; 42; 43; 44; 45; 46; 47

R

raisins; 29; 154; 168
red capsicum; 61
rhubarb; 147
rice; 51; 100; 101; 107; 109; 114; 120; 144; 155; 189; 246
ricotta; 61; 70; 122
romaine; 95
rosemary; 94; 177; 222

S

sage; 104; 147
salmon; 33; 34; 157; 158; 159; 163; 166; 173; 175; 178; 185; 186; 193; 194; 200
salsa; 7; 153; 201
sausage; 94; 101

scallions; 141
sesame oil; 51; 102; 109
sesame seeds; 127; 188
shallot; 36; 103; 133; 148; 149; 185
sherry; 152
shrimp; 73; 87; 113; 114; 115; 116; 164; 167; 181; 183; 184; 189; 194
sour cream; 67; 76; 86; 99; 120
soy sauce; 53; 79; 82; 88; 91; 101; 102; 106; 115; 124; 127; 131; 139; 144; 146; 152; 159; 175
spinach; 41; 42; 47; 97; 125; 194
squash; 71; 83
squid; 192
steak; 30; 39; 74; 92; 102; 111; 188
strawberries; 125; 231; 238
sugar; 29; 143; 147; 148; 154; 175; 226; 228; 231; 233; 235; 236; 237; 238; 240; 241; 242; 244; 245; 246; 247; 248; 250

T

Tabasco sauce; 214
tarragon; 71; 125; 152; 191
tentacles; 192
thyme; 9; 50; 83; 100; 119; 133; 135; 137; 138; 149; 171; 172; 224
tofu; 18; 22; 23; 40
tomatoes; 10; 68; 78; 83; 85; 88; 100; 105; 134; 143; 177; 183; 198; 200; 207; 209; 215; 220; 221; 222
tortillas; 46; 56; 70; 86; 201
tuna; 188; 197; 198; 199
turkey; 46; 143
turmeric; 50; 66; 170

V

vanilla; 29; 64; 208; 230; 235; 238; 239; 240; 241; 242; 244; 246; 247; 250

W

watercress; 179
white vinegar; 84; 240
white wine; 87; 152
wine; 144; 148; 191
Worcestershire sauce; 32; 91; 97

Y

yogurt; 154; 173

Z

zucchini; 36; 71; 152; 153; 156; 200; 203

g. sso paso mm	Kern fond int. núcleo ⌀ mm	trap mèche broca ⌀ mm
	2.46	2.5
0.5	3.24	3
0.7	4.13	
0.8	4.92	
1	6.65	

APPENDIX WITH CONVERSION MEASURE

WEIGHTS	
IMPERIAL	METRIC
½ oz.	15 g
¾ oz.	20 g
1 oz.	30 g
2 oz.	60 g
3 oz.	85 g
16 oz. = 1 pound = 435 g	
1 oz. = 28.35 g | 1 g = 0.035 oz.	

COMMON INGREDIENTS

1 CUP	IMPERIAL	METRIC
Flour	5 oz.	140 g
Almonds	4 oz.	110 g
Uncooked Rice	6½ oz.	190 g
Brown Sugar	6½ oz.	185 g
Raisins	7 oz.	200 g
Grated Cheese	4 oz.	115 g

LIQUIDS

CUPS	METRIC	PINT	QUART
¼	60 ml	-	-
½	125 ml	-	-
-	150 ml	¼	-
-	200 ml	-	-
1	250 ml	½	-
-	300 ml	-	-
-	400 ml	-	-
2	500 ml	-	-
-	950 ml	-	1

OVEN TEMPS

°F	°C
250	120
275	140
300	150
325	170
350	180
375	190
400	200

SPOONS

LIQUID		DRY	
¼ tsp.	1.25 ml	¼ tsp.	1.1 g
½ tsp.	2.5 ml	½ tsp.	2.3 g
1 tsp.	5 ml	1 tsp.	4.7 g
¼ tbsp.	3.75 ml	¼ tbsp.	3.5 g
½ tbsp.	7.5 ml	½ tbsp.	7.1 g
1 tbsp.	15 ml	1 tbsp.	14.3 g

RECIPE INDEX

BREAKFAST 17

1. Air Fried Asparagus 17
2. Air Fried Sandwich 17
3. Amazing Crab Breakfast 17
4. Asparagus Frittata 17
5. Bacon and Ham Mix 17
6. Bell Pepper Breakfast Mix 18
7. Black Beans with Eggs 18
8. Broccoli Breakfast Mix 18
9. Broccoli Quiche 18
10. Carrot Mixed Chicken 19
11. Cheese Burger Patties 19
12. Chicken Mix 19
13. Chicken with Cheese 19
14. Chicken with Orange Taste 19
15. Dates and Millet Pudding 20
16. Delicious Shrimp 20
17. Delicious Tofu and Mushrooms 20
18. Dill Eggs 20
19. Egg Sauce Breakfast 20
20. Eggs with Onion 21
21. Fish and Bread 21
22. Fluffy Egg 21
23. French Toast Delight 21
24. Garlic and Cheese Bread Rolls 21
25. Hearty Breakfast with Bacon 23
26. Lettuce Mixed Breakfast 23
27. Meat Patties for Breakfast 23
28. Muffin Mix Breakfast 23
29. Oatmeal Breakfast 23
30. Potato Mix Breakfast 24

31.	Quick Eggs	24
32.	Rarebit Air Fried Egg	24
33.	Salmon Breakfast with Carrot Mix	24
34.	Salmon Mixed Eggs	24
35.	Scrambled Eggs	25
36.	Shallot Mix	25
37.	Simple Bacon and Eggs	25
38.	Simple Bacon	25
39.	Simple Breakfast	25
40.	Smoked Air Fried Tofu	26
41.	Spinach Breakfast Parcels	26
42.	Spinach Mushroom Mix	26
43.	Steak Strips	26
44.	Thai Style Omelette	27
45.	Tofu for Breakfast	27
46.	Turkey Burrito	27
47.	Veggie Mix	27

SNACKS & SIDE DISHES 29

48.	Air Fried Cheeseburger	29
49.	Avocado Fries	29
50.	Avocado Sticks	29
51.	Cauliflower Rice	29
52.	Chia Seeds Snack	30
53.	Chicken Legs	30
54.	Chickpeas Snack	30
55.	Coconut Cream Potatoes	30
56.	Corn Tortilla Chips	30
57.	Corn with Lime and Cheese	30
58.	Corncobs	31
59.	Cornmeal Mix Snack	31
60.	Creamy Air Fried Potato	31
61.	Delicious Muffin Snack	31
62.	Grilled Cheese Delight	31
63.	Hasselback Potatoes	33
64.	Nutella Mix Snack	33

65.	Nuts Mix Snack	33
66.	Puff Pastry Appetizer	33
67.	Spring Onion Mix Snack	33
68.	Sundried Tomatoes Snack	34
69.	Sweet Potato Fries	34
70.	Tortillas with Banana	34
71.	Yellow Squash and Zucchinis	34

BEEF, PORK & LAMB .... Errore. Il segnalibro non è definito.

72.	Amazing Beef Balls	36
73.	Bacon Mixed	36
74.	Bacon with Mustard	36
75.	Bacon-Wrapped Hot Dog	36
76.	Beef and Pork Mix	36
77.	Beef Breast Pieces with Celery	37
78.	Beef Loaf with Black Olives	37
79.	Beef Mix Carrot	37
80.	Beef Steak Delight	37
81.	Beef Steak with Tomato Soup	38
82.	Beef Strips with Snow Peas and Mushrooms	38
83.	Beef Stuffed Squash	38
84.	Beef with Arugula	38
85.	Beef with Cheese Mix	38
86.	Beef with Corn Kernels	39
87.	Beef with Linguine	39
88.	Beef with Mushrooms	39
89.	Beef with Mushrooms and Onions	39
90.	Beef with Potatoes	39
91.	Beef Worcestershire	40
92.	Buttered Striploin Steak	40
93.	Cheeseburgers Air Fried	40
94.	Comforting Sausage Casserole	40
95.	Crispy Pork Chop Salad	42
96.	Easy Juicy Pork Chops	42
97.	Ground Beef with Spinach Leaves	42
98.	Grounded Beef with Bacon	42

99.	Grounded Beef with Pork and Veal	43
100.	Grounded Beef with Rice	43
101.	Grounded Pork with Carrots and Rice	43
102.	Maple Syrup Mix Beef	43
103.	Mediterranean Steaks and Scallops	43
104.	Pork Chops and Sage Sauce	44
105.	Pork with Black Olives	44
106.	Pork with Honey Mix	44
107.	Pork with White Rice	44
108.	Provencal Pork	44
109.	Quick Beef	45
110.	Red Meat Delight	45
111.	Reverse Seared Ribeye	45
112.	Scallops with Beef Special	45
113.	Shrimp and Beef with Lettuce	45
114.	Shrimps and Red Meat Mix	46
115.	Shrimps with Honey and Beef	46
116.	Simply Beef and Shrimp	46

POULTRY .... Errore. Il segnalibro non è definito.

117.	Buffalo Chicken Meatballs	48
118.	Buffalo Wings	48
119.	Carrots and Chicken	48
120.	Cheese and Broccoli Chicken	48
121.	Chicken and Black Olives Sauce	49
122.	Chicken and Bow Pasta	49
123.	Chicken and Capers	49
124.	Chicken and Chestnuts Mix	49
125.	Chicken and Spinach Salad	50
126.	Chicken Breast with Marsala	50
127.	Chicken Kabobs	50
128.	Chicken Parmesan Cutlets	50
129.	Chicken Tenders	51
130.	Chicken Thighs with Stock	51
131.	Chicken Wings	51
132.	Chicken Wings with Hot Sauce	51

133.	Chicken with Apple	52
134.	Chicken with Black Beans	52
135.	Chicken with Buttermilk	52
136.	Chicken with Garlic	52
137.	Chicken with Lemon Juice	52
138.	Chicken with Lemon Zest	54
139.	Chicken with Mushrooms	54
140.	Chicken with Potatoes	54
141.	Chicken with Scallions	54
142.	Chicken with Spices	54
143.	Chicken Garlic Turkey	55
144.	Chinese Duck Legs	55
145.	Creamy Stock	55
146.	Crispy Chicken Wings	55
147.	Duck and Cherries	56
148.	Duck and Plum Sauce	56
149.	Duck with Balsamic Vinegar	56
150.	Honey Duck Breast	56
151.	Jalapeno and Avocado Chicken	56
152.	Marinated Duck Breasts	57
153.	Mexican Chicken Breast	57
154.	Roasted Chicken with Mayo	57
155.	Tomato Sauce Chicken	57
156.	White Beans with Chicken	58

FISH & SEAFOOD 60

157.	Almond Pesto Salmon	60
158.	Amazing Salmon Fillets	60
159.	Asian Salmon	60
160.	Black Beans with Ham and Salmon	60
161.	Black Beans with Mackerel	61
162.	Cajun Salmon	61
163.	Celery and Salmon Fillets	61
164.	Chickpeas and Shrimp	61
165.	Chickpeas with Crab	61
166.	Cilantro Lime Baked Salmon	62

167.	Coconut Shrimp	62
168.	Cod Fillets with Fennel and Grapes Salad	62
169.	Cod Fillets with Squash	62
170.	Cod Steaks with Plum Sauce	63
171.	Cod with Celery Stalk	63
172.	Cod with Pearl Onions	63
173.	Creamy Salmon	63
174.	Crumbled Fish	63
175.	Flavored Air Fried Salmon	64
176.	Foil-Packet Lobster Tail	64
177.	Halibut and Sun-Dried Tomatoes Mix	64
178.	Hawaiian Salmon	64
179.	Honey Sea Bass	66
180.	Juicy Salmon and Asparagus Parcels	66
181.	Lemon Garlic Shrimp	66
182.	Mackerel with Sweet Potatoes	66
183.	Mushrooms with Shrimps	66
184.	Quick and Easy Shrimp	67
185.	Salmon and Lemon Relish	67
186.	Salmon and Orange Marmalade	67
187.	Salmon Patties	67
188.	Sweet Cashew Sticks	67
189.	Shrimp and Cauliflower	68
190.	Simple Buttery Cod	68
191.	Snapper Fillets and Veggies	68
192.	Squid and Guacamole	68
193.	Steamed Salmon with Dill Sauce	69
194.	Stuffed Salmon	69
195.	Super-Simple Scallops	69
196.	Swordfish and Mango Salsa	69
197.	Tuna Fish with Squash	70
198.	Tuna Fish with Tomato Paste	70
199.	Tuna Puff Pastry	70
200.	Zucchini with Salmon Fillets	70

PLANT BASED 72

    201. Beans Burrito 72

    202. Bell Pepper Oatmeal 72

    203. Black Beans Mix Soup 72

    204. Black Eyed Peas 72

    205. Broccoli and Mushrooms Mix 73

    206. Broccoli Mix 73

    207. Brussels Sprouts and Tomatoes 73

    208. Chia Pudding 73

    209. Chicken and Mushrooms 73

    210. Chicken Tomato Sauce 74

    211. Crispy French Fries 74

    212. Frying Potatoes with Butter 74

    213. Homemade French Fries 74

    214. Hot Cabbage Mix 74

    215. Mediterranean Chickpeas 74

    216. Portobello Mini Pizzas 76

    217. Roasted Broccoli Salad 76

    218. Spinach Cheese Pie 76

    219. Sweet Potatoes and Corn 76

    220. Tomato Frittata 76

    221. Tomatoes and Basil Mix 76

    222. Tomatoes Salad 77

    223. Vegan Cheese Sandwich 77

    224. Veggie Broth with Cauliflower 77

    225. White Mushrooms Mix 77

DESSERTS 79

    226. Apple Chips 79

    227. Apples and Wine Sauce 79

    228. Apples Mix Dessert 79

    229. Black Cherries Dessert 79

    230. Brioche Bread 80

    231. Cake with Strawberries Cream 80

    232. Chocolate Banana 80

    233. Chocolate Chips 80

234.	Chocolate Mixed Cocoa	80
235.	Coconut Mix Dessert	81
236.	Delicious Buttercream	81
237.	Honey Cake	81
238.	Kiwi and Strawberry Mix	81
239.	Oats and Blueberries Mix	83
240.	Pecans Filled Dessert	83
241.	Raspberry Jam Delight	83
242.	Red Velvet Cake	83
243.	Saltine Crackers Mix	84
244.	Simple Cake	84
245.	Simple Sweet Sheets	84
246.	Soft Rice	84
247.	Sweet Potato Dessert	84
248.	Vermicelli Mix	85
249.	Walnut Milk	85
250.	White Chocolate	85

Made in the USA
Monee, IL
05 May 2021